## TRUE OR FALSE?

A fever of 104°F or higher is always an emergency.
　Answer: FALSE

Childproofing will guarantee your child's safety.
　Answer: FALSE

Baby aspirin is always safe for children.
　Answer: FALSE

Cough and cold medicines are neither safe nor effective
in children two and under.
　Answer: TRUE

Kids can get bronchitis.
　Answer: FALSE

Most cases of pink eye don't require antibiotics.
　Answer: TRUE

An ear infection requires emergency treatment.
　Answer: FALSE

If your baby produces only one stool a week, he/she
is constipated.
　Answer: FALSE

Antibiotics are not effective against a virus.
　Answer: TRUE

### IF YOUR KID EATS THIS BOOK, EVERYTHING WILL STILL BE OKAY

#### How to Know if Your Child's Injury or Illness Is *Really* an Emergency

# if your kid eats this book, everything will still be okay

## How to Know if Your Child's Injury or Illness Is *Really* an Emergency

### Lara Zibners, MD

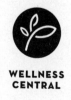

**WELLNESS CENTRAL**

NEW YORK    BOSTON

Wellness Central
Hachette Book Group
237 Park Avenue
New York, NY 10017

Visit our Web site at www.HachetteBookGroup.com.

Wellness Central is an imprint of Grand Central Publishing.
The Wellness Central name and logo are trademarks of Hachette Book Group, Inc.

Printed in the United States of America

First Edition: June 2009
10 9 8 7 6 5 4 3 2 1

Library of Congress Cataloging-in-Publication Data

Zibners, Lara.
    If your kid eats this book, everything will still be okay : how to know if your child's injury or illness is really an emergency / Lara Zibners.—1st ed.
        p. cm.
    Includes index.
    Summary: "A funny and practical guide to knowing when your child's predicament is actually worth panicking about—from a former New York City Emergency Room pediatrician"—Provided by the publisher.
    ISBN 978-0-446-50880-3
    1. Pediatric emergencies—Popular works. 2. Children—Wounds and injuries—Popular works. I. Title.
RJ370.Z53.2009
618.92'0025—dc22                    2008044504

Book design and text composition by Anne Ricigliano

# acknowledgments

This little project could never have happened without the time, dedication, and, frankly, blind support of so many people in my past, present, and, hopefully, future.

To my high school AP Biology teacher, Mr. Steven Ruggiero, who listened to me lament the excruciating boredom of scientific writing and told me that he had faith that someday I would be the one to find a way to make it interesting, I hope I did.

To every teacher who taught me how to become a scientist, nurtured my writings, or just helped me believe in myself, thank you.

To my friends, colleagues, and mentors who taught me the art of medicine, I try to remember those lessons every day.

To the nurses and staff who gently corralled an occasionally arrogant young doctor and taught me to respect you, I remember that always.

To my parents and sisters, who have unquestionably supported and proudly suffered through years of my never-ending education and the complete self-absorption that naturally accompanies such pursuits, thank you for still liking me.

To my friends who have listened to me talk about "writing a book" and actually believed it would happen, thank you for your senseless enthusiasm.

To my agents, Jeff Kleinman and Erin Niumata, and all the fabulous folks at Folio Literary Management, thanks for taking a leap on a total unknown and in the process becoming such dear friends.

To the people at Hachette Book Group, especially my editor, Natalie Kaire, thank you for believing that a doctor can also write and for pouring so much energy into this venture.

To my medical advisory review panel, Drs. John Fortney, Adam Vella, Daniel Cohen, and James Naprawa, thank you for your brains, time, and love.

And a final thank-you to my husband, Gernot, because it was your idea and we all know it.

# contents

## 4  Seeing and Hearing: The Eyes and Ears    76

## 5  Bite and Sniff: The Nose, Mouth, and Throat    90

# introduction

## What's This Book about Anyway?

Are you the kind of parent who panics every time your kid hits his head or wipes away a drop of snot? Or are you the parent handing a hemophiliac four-year-old a box cutter? Maybe you don't actually have any kids and just like dropping fascinating tidbits of information at dinner parties. Whatever the case, this book has got something for you. What would happen if your child ate the decorative pebbles in the fish tank? Actually, probably nothing. But a teaspoon of what liquid lurking in your medicine cabinet could kill a room full of toddlers? How do you know if a kid is dehydrated or not? Sick with pneumonia or just a cold? Has appendicitis or just a bellyache?

This book is not about the basics of child care such as bathing, diapering, and feeding. There are many wonderful books out there that already cover these topics. Instead, this book is a regurgitation, if you will, of all the midnight conversations I've had with stressed and anxious parents. As a pediatrician with specialized training in pediatric emergency medicine, I have expertise in treating ill and injured kids. It's what I love to do. However, somewhere along the way I started thinking, "Hey, there should be a book about this." Twenty-five million kids in the United States are taken to the ER each year, and more than 50 percent of these visits may be unnecessary. The intent of this book is to help parents avoid the stress and expense of a potentially needless visit to the doctor or ER. How are parents supposed to know when a kid needs to be seen by his pediatrician and when he just needs chicken soup? What should they do if someone drops the baby? If his sister puts household bleach in his bottle, is he going to be okay?

## IT'S NOT REALLY A ROOM

TV has turned *ER* into a household term, yet this rankles many emergency physicians. The emergency room is not a "room," but is an entire department consisting of many little rooms and an entire team of doctors, nurses, and other staff members. The proper term is *emergency department*, or *ED*. However, since *ER* is what you're probably most familiar with, I'll refer to it as such. But be forewarned that any doctor working in an "ER" is likely to correct your terminology.

For many parents, fear and worry quickly replace the overwhelming joy and excitement that accompany the arrival of a child. What a responsibility. If you listen to the media, it is amazing that anyone survives childhood at all. A kid gets the flu and dies the next day. A child falls from an escalator at the mall. An alligator stalks dogs and children in a residential neighborhood.

How does a parent keep any perspective amid this storm of terror? Bad things can happen. But tragedies like these are, fortunately, rare. Kids are pretty resilient. The intent of this book is to arm you with the information you need to know to help determine if your kid needs medical attention and what simple steps you can take to keep him safe and well. By helping you decide if your kid's ailment may be an emergency, hopefully you will be more easily able to sit back, relax, and enjoy your little one. After all, isn't that why you signed on for this adventure in the first place?

However, please remember that this is just a guide. And remember: This book is not intended to be a substitute for specific medical advice. You know your kid better than

## AFTER-HOURS DOCTORING

Most pediatricians would prefer that, in the absence of a life-threatening emergency, they be called before their patients are taken to the ER. Even at two o'clock in the morning. This ensures not only that patients don't make unnecessary trips to the hospital, but also that the doctor has the opportunity to call ahead and speak with the ER team, so that they are expecting the patient and have some basic background information. Don't think that you are helping your doctor by not waking her up or bothering her on the weekend. She honestly wants to know what is happening to her patient. That said, I do know that not all doctors' offices offer after-hours services. In some places I indicate that you should call the doctor before making any decisions, but if you are unable to reach your kid's pediatrician or are in any way worried that you cannot wait for a return call, go ahead and come on into the ER.

## CALLING THE ER YOURSELF

The American College of Emergency Physicians strictly advises against giving any information to patients over the phone. Doctors and nurses in the ER cannot and should not give medical advice over the phone.

anyone, and I'm not sitting with you and your kid in your living room. If there is ever *any doubt* that your child is in need of medical attention, *don't hesitate* to call your pediatrician or 911. Your pediatrician should be your first line of defense against rushing out the door at midnight, and this book will help you decide whether it is worth waking her up. And if you do, and she says you need to go to the hospital, I'll prepare you for what will happen once you get there.

I have done my very best to make sure the information in here is as accurate and up to date as possible, enlisting a few of my friends and colleagues, all of whom are pediatricians specializing in pediatric emergency medicine, to make sure that I wasn't speaking in tongues. When there is *any* doubt, please, consult your pediatrician. Don't hesitate for a

## GO LOOK THEM UP

Drs. John Fortney, Adam Vella, James Naprawa, and Daniel Cohen: my medical advisory review panel. Experts in Pediatric Emergency Medicine. The guys who read through my late-night rantings to make sure I wasn't saying anything too off base. If you happen upon any one of them, give him a big smooch for me.

second to alert Emergency Medical Services in case of an emergency. And if you don't know if it's really an emergency, err on the side of caution. Please. Your child's health and safety are at stake.

That said, let's get going.

## Dr. Zibners's Rules

Before we really begin, let me share with you a few of my personal rules when it comes to deciding if a kid is truly ill or injured:

- A crying child has an airway and is conscious.
- When "everything hurts," probably nothing is really broken.
- Babies and toddlers don't fake pain.
- Never trust a toddler. (Who knows what they ate/stuck in their nose/fed the baby?)
- Always trust your gut.

### How to Use This Book

As you read this book, you'll find little asides that point out interesting tidbits of information or alert you to common myths about childhood illnesses. In a few places, you'll find "Warning!" notes to let you know of steps you can take to prevent injury or illness. "Emergency!" notations should alert you to the fact that your pediatrician likely needs to be called, even at midnight. And finally, "911!" signs will tell you when to stop reading, pick up the phone, and call for an ambulance.

## THE MEDICINE CABINET ESSENTIALS

### *Dosages*

Always check with your pediatrician about the appropriate dose or a medication for your child. If your kid is particularly chunky or petite, the "age-recommended" dosing on the box may not be appropriate. Also, many over-the-counter medicines have labels that recommend a dose at the very bottom of an appropriate dose range, meaning the amount of medicine *might* be slightly too little to see a desired effect. But this applies only to *some* medicine, so don't up the dosages yourself without checking.

### *Age Appropriateness*

Always check with your doctor before giving pain or fever medication to an infant less than three months of age.

### *What to Keep in the Cabinet*

- Acetaminophen (Tylenol), infant or child: While great for treating pain and fever, be aware that acetaminophen can be very toxic in an overdose. The infant formulations are much more concentrated than the children's, so be very, very careful when measuring out an age- and weight-appropriate dose. This medication is also available in a rectal suppository, a great thing to have on hand if your kid is vomiting or refusing medication.

- Ibuprofen (Motrin or Advil), infant or child: With the added bonus of treating swelling, or inflammation, in addition to pain and fever, ibuprofen is sometimes the better choice. Again, the infant and child formulations are of extremely different concentrations so be very careful. Ibuprofen is not officially approved for kids less than six months of age.

- Diphenhydramine (Benadryl) oral liquid (not cream): The first-line treatment for an allergic reaction, itching, or hives, diphenhydramine is quite safe but can make a child sleepy. Some kids have the opposite response and go crazy. Check with your doctor before giving diphenhydramine to a baby younger than a year.

- Antibiotic ointment (e.g., Neosporin): Good to have on hand for cuts and scratches to prevent infection and promote healing, antibiotic ointment should generally be applied two to three times a day until a wound is better.

- Diaper rash cream: Any good diaper rash cream should contain a protecting "barrier" cream and a metal salt, such as magnesium or aluminum. Not just for diaper rash, the cream will soothe any sore areas, such as a little bottom that is raw and chafed from several episodes of diarrhea.

- Petroleum jelly (Vaseline): Good for protecting sore areas of skin and for dissolving superglue between body parts. Also it's a great moisturizer for really dry skin when slathered on just after a bath.

- 1% hydrocortisone cream: Usually available as 0.5% or 1% in over-the-counter preparations, hydrocortisone helps with the itching of bug bites, allergic reactions, and eczema. However, steroid creams should be applied only sparingly, only to the skin being treated, and never in the diaper area or skin that otherwise can't breathe properly. The cream should be applied up to two times a day and *only* for up to seven days without doctor supervision.

- Sunscreen (SPF 15 at the *minimum*): Sunscreen should always be handy and applied at least thirty minutes before going outside. Reapply every two hours or after getting wet or sweaty. Sunscreen should only be applied very sparingly to babies under six months and only on areas that aren't protected by clothing or shade.

- Adhesive bandages, an assortment of sizes and shapes.

- Elastic bandages: Good for wrapping a mild sprain, or keeping a difficult-to-cover wound clean, elastic bandages

can also be used to strap an ice pack to an injured limb
or help to apply a makeshift splint in an emergency.

■ Ice packs: Formal ice packs are great to keep in the
freezer, although a bag of frozen peas will work just as
well. Ice packs should *never* be applied directly to the skin.
Always keep wrapped in a towel and apply for twenty minutes at a time as tolerated to treat swelling and pain.

## What Not to Keep in the Cabinet

Aspirin, even baby aspirin, is usually not recommended at all for
children except in very special circumstances as it has been
associated with a rare condition that can cause liver and brain
problems. Cough and cold medicines *don't* work, and many will
make kids either sleepy or very irritable. Last, anything that is
not indicated for children, such as adult formulations of pain
medicine, diarrhea or indigestion medications, or anything that
does not give specific dosing instructions for a child should
*never* be given to one without first speaking to your physician.

# ten fingers . . . eleven toes?

## A Guide to the Newborn's Body, Behaviors, and Symptoms

The balloons are in the driveway, the cigars passed to all the neighbors. Now you are sitting in the living room, staring at the basket in the corner, sizing up your tiny opponent. Rather than sitting there, looking shell shocked and petrified, go pick little Johnny up, bring him over to the couch, strip off his fuzzy bunting, and dig right in. Is he supposed to have that spot? Why is his head shaped that way? Can he see you? Let's start this book by getting to know the newborn and making sure that all those things that are guaranteed to freak you out at 2 a.m. have been dealt with so you can move on. Most of your

### WHAT IS A NEWBORN?

In proper medical terms, *newborn* refers to an infant between zero and twenty-eight days old. While four weeks seems like a very short period of time, in the baby world exceptional things can happen. In one month, a little one goes from a curled-up lump with a slightly misshapen head to something almost resembling the creature commonly known as a "baby."

concerns can be found in other parts of this book, but here we'll touch on those that are particularly common in newborns *and* particularly prone to causing panic.

> **WARNING!**
>
> A fever in a newborn is considered an urgency. With few exceptions, this is the only time that fever alone, regardless of any other symptoms, demands a phone call and an evaluation. A fever in a newborn baby is defined as 38°C or 100.4°F.

## Dropping the Baby

Let's just get this one out of the way. You've dropped the baby. Maybe you fell asleep and she rolled down your leg and onto the carpet. Maybe you turned your back "for just a second" and there she was, screaming on the floor. Stop, take a big breath. Don't panic. Most babies survive their first experience with gravity just fine. Here's what you do need to know. If the baby is screaming and mad, moving everything, and looking at you with evil in her eyes, carefully feel her head, her back, and her arms and legs, and if everything seems okay, pick her up and turn to "Falls," on page 262. Call your doctor to let her know what happened. Without any external evidence of injury and with a moving, screaming, and purple-mad baby, most likely everything is fine.

> **911!**
>
> If the baby falls and is not moving or crying, if she has a very weak cry or seems not alert or her color seems pale or blue, *call 911.* Don't move the baby unless she is in immediate danger of falling farther.

## How Far Is Too Far?

The rule in pediatric emergency medicine is "Under three months, over three feet," meaning that an infant younger than twelve weeks who tumbles more than thirty-six inches may need a head CT to rule out any serious injury. You should probably call your doctor.

## Ten Little Fingers, Ten Little Toes

As soon as the nurse left the room, you unwrapped that blanket and checked to make sure he had ten fingers and ten toes, didn't you? What if you found eleven? It happens. No big deal. Extra fingers and toes tend to run in families, so check out Grandpa's feet next time you're at the beach. Some of these little digits are just small growths of skin and others have little bones. Either way, they come off pretty easily. Some physicians will tie them with a suture (after confirming the absence of any bone) until they literally just fall right off. Others prefer to have them removed by a surgeon. Just don't forget to warn him before he counts the toes of his own child someday.

## Deep Breath In . . .

Newborns sputter. They gag. They turn red. They cough and sneeze. If you are worried about the way she is breathing, refer to Chapter 2, and if in doubt, call your doctor immediately. But you should know about this funky little newborn quirk called periodic breathing. They breathe really fast for a few seconds and then pause. It comes in little waves, especially when they are sleeping: normal breathing, really fast breathing, pause, normal breathing, really fast breathing, pause.

These pauses are frightening, but last only a couple of seconds and then baby starts breathing again, all on her own. As long as the pauses are only a few seconds long, the baby *never changes color*, and begins breathing again with no help from you, this is normal. Completely normal. Babies have immature brains and the part that controls breathing will eventually mature and she will start breathing in a more regular pattern.

## From Head to Toe

Now let us start at the top and work our way slowly down. It's how we were taught to do physician exams in medical school and it seems to work. This way I can try to systematically assure you that what you've found is normal, point out some things that you may not have noticed, and help to avoid a bleary-eyed 3 a.m. freak-out.

### The Noggin

Take his hat off. Now look for the little scab where the fetal monitor was attached. If you see new blisters forming or the wound starts to look infected, give your doctor a call. Otherwise keep reading.

*The Soft Spot.* Have you ever wondered why a baby horse can stand up a few minutes after birth and within a few days is running around the farm like nothing happened while a human baby just lies there, day in and day out, staring at the ceiling, not even making rudimentary attempts to walk? It's because we're smarter than horses. And I don't mean because babies know that, by lying there, people will cater to them and they have to do essentially no work at all. I mean that our brains are bigger than the brains of most animals. Our heads are also larger in proportion to the rest of our bodies. So, in order for us to squeeze ourselves down the birth canal, we have to be born while we are still relatively small and immature. Hence, the helpless baby. Because our brains are going to continue to grow after we are born, the bones of our skull must be able to move and grow accordingly. Hence the "soft spot."

In medical terms, the "soft spot" is called the anterior fontanel. It is the meeting point of two bones of the skull, which will over time grow together, fusing into a solid skull. There are actually two fontanels at birth, but the one found on the front half of the tiptop of the head is the one you can most easily feel. Soft spots vary in size considerably and will most likely get bigger before closing up. Some babies have soft spots that are flat while others seem to bulge up a bit. In some newborns the bones may seem to overlap a bit and that is okay too. If you are at all worried that the soft spot is abnormal, call your doctor, but if your baby is behaving like a normal newborn, it's probably fine.

Don't worry about poking his brain out either. You can run a hairbrush over the soft spot and you won't hurt anything. There is a whole lot of nice thick skin and muscle and other good stuff protecting the contents of his skull.

**He's a Conehead!** There is a reason we put hats on little babies immediately after birth and it's not because they might catch cold. After spending several hours squeezing his way down the old birth canal, there is a good chance that his head will have "molded" and look rather misshapen for several days. A bit of swelling over parts of the scalp is also to be expected. This usually goes down over the first two to three days of life. Some babies actually develop some bleeding under the scalp (not on the brain!) during the birthing process that we call a cephalohematoma. That is a big word for "bruised scalp." Typically this occurs after a prolonged or difficult labor. Unless unusually large, these also pose no issues for the little peanut. The swelling may grow over the first couple of days and then take a few weeks to resolve. As the collection of blood dissolves, it may feel either hard like an eggshell or very soft and gushy. Both are normal. If you are concerned, just ask your pediatrician to take a look at the baby's head. And then put his hat back on.

*If You Can Get His Eyes Open.* At birth a baby's eyesight is good enough to see your face but gets a bit fuzzy when looking across the room at the TV. Color vision gradually appears by two to four months. In other words, if Dad is trying to convince the family that the brand-new 28-inch HD TV in your living room is for the baby, he should come up with a better story. If you are trying to see what color the baby's eyes are, try holding him upright. Newborns are loath to open up when lying down, wrapped up all cozy in a blanket.

Now that they are open, don't be alarmed if you see a large red area on the white part of the eyeball. This is called a subconjunctival, or scleral, hemorrhage, which is simply a broken blood vessel overlying the sclera, or white part, of the eye. Coughing vigorously, vomiting, or laughing hysterically are common causes of subconjunctival hemorrhages. Increased pressure in your face can make a little vessel burst. Having your face squashed along the walls of a birth canal can certainly do it. It will go away by itself within a couple of weeks. Don't fret.

*Natal Teeth.* Rarely, some babies are born with teeth. Even more rarely will a newborn have a tooth pop through the gum in the first few weeks after birth. These are usually rudimentary little teeth, not true teeth, and most will be removed shortly after birth. These teeth would fall out on their own but we pull them because most are very wobbly and not securely fastened to the gums. They also may cause some irritation to the tongue and lips. Just point them out to your physician if he failed to notice them in the nursery.

## The Torso

*The Wishbone.* Do you know what the equivalent in humans is to the wishbone in a turkey? The clavicles. These are the bones at the top of the chest that help create the frame from which your arms hang. Sometimes during a more difficult delivery, one of these bones may break. If not noticed immediately after birth, you may later detect a small amount of swelling or feel a hard bump along one of the clavicles. These bones heal very well and this bump will eventually go away. This is a pretty common injury and does not in any way mean that the doctor was too aggressive during the birth.

*The Waiter's Tip.* In the same way that the clavicle can be broken during delivery, the bundle of nerves that start in the neck and run under the clavicle and into the armpit might also become injured during the birth process. Depending on which nerves are injured, a baby may have weakness of all or part of the arm. In many cases, a baby's arm will hang limply at his side when he's propped upward, with the hand facing backward as if waiting for a $20 tip after showing you to your seat. Absolutely any sign of weakness in the arm should be called to the attention of your doctor as some of these injuries may require further evaluation or repair.

*The Breastbone.* Some babies have a breastbone, or sternum, that caves inward (pectus excavatum), while others bow outward (pectus carinatum). Either way, newborns' chests are very soft and mobile and everything may seem quite exaggerated at this stage. Don't worry if you see ribs and bones, and everything seems to pull this way and that. At the very end of the sternum is a little bump, called the xiphoid process. This is just the tip of the sternum, but because babies and kids are still growing, it isn't fully attached yet to the main bone, making it seem more prominent and a lot of parents mistake it for a tumor or other abnormal growth. It's not.

**Breast Bumps.** Try to remember how incredibly hormonal moms feel when pregnant. And then remember that a little one was sitting inside this sea of hormones. So it's no wonder that babies can have estrogen and testosterone levels rivaling that of a teenager for a period of time after birth. Many babies will develop some swelling of the breasts or occasionally have some milky discharge from the nipples. This is a result of hormones and not true breast development. As the hormone levels fall to normal, there will be no more discharge and the breasts will return to normal baby size. Some babies will actually develop an infection in the breast, resulting in redness of the skin, more swelling on one side than the other, or a foul-appearing discharge. If any of these symptoms develop, call your pediatrician immediately.

**Supernummary Nipples.** Speaking of breast issues, some babies have extra nipples. These are called supernummary nipples but you may have heard them referred to as "witches' tits." During early embryonic development, we all have several rudimentary nipples that develop in a row on the front of the developing torso. Normally all but the uppermost disappear. You don't have to do anything about this, but if you are worried that he's going to get teased endlessly in the locker room, a plastic surgeon will be able to remove the extra little nubbin later.

*Belly Buttons.* Belly buttons. Some people have "outies"; some have "innies." Some are filled with lint and others are decorated with metal studs. The medical term is the umbilicus. Most of us don't give them a lot of thought. But early on, at the very beginning, when Daddy is strong-armed into sawing through this life-giving yet surprisingly tough and rubbery appendage that stretches strangely from the middle of your baby, the "umbilical cord" becomes every parent's worry. Along with wiping away spit-up and changing diapers, caring for The Cord becomes part of caring for baby. And with every passing day, Mom and Dad can find new reasons to worry about their little one. A small amount of oozing blood is completely normal. A slightly goopy and gelatinous consistency to the base of the cord is also normal. You simply need to make sure that any cord care regimen your pediatrician has recommended, such as applying rubbing alcohol, actually involves the base of the cord that remains attached to the baby. Repeatedly wiping the already dried-out piece sticking two inches away from baby is an exercise in futility.

## HOW LONG?

Most umbilical stumps will dry up and fall off by two to three weeks of age. Don't pull on the cord, even if it is hanging by a thread. Let it fall off on its own.

The following are absolutely not normal: Any foul-smelling or discolored drainage from the newborn's belly button warrants an urgent evaluation. Any redness spreading onto the belly is also an absolute urgency. (A small amount of pink tissue right at the center of the umbilicus is normal healing tissue, however.) Also, please let your doctor know if there is any persistent drainage of any type coming from the umbilicus after the cord has fallen off.

**Sacral Dimple.** Now, flip him over and look at his back. Pay special attention to the area just above his little baby bottom. A tuft of hair or little dimple should be pointed out to your doctor, but it's not an emergency. Abnormalities at the base of the spine are quite common and infrequently significant but can rarely signify an underlying problem with the lower spine. Your pediatrician may decide to evaluate this further with special X-ray studies, but not in the middle of the night.

## In the Diaper

**Urine Output: Dry Diapers.** New parents are often advised to keep track of the "outputs" deposited in little Marge's diapers. While this is especially important for breastfed infants, when we are not sure of their actual intake during the first several days of life, some parents exhibit a tendency to become, how shall I say this, obsessed. Some parents actually go so far as to carry a small notebook filled with detailed information such as how many milliliters little Marge drank at 1:32 a.m. and how many grams of output were received at 2:08 a.m. If you are so sleep deprived that you are afraid you will forget who little Marge is, let alone what she ate and when she pooped, then please get yourself a notebook and follow suit. We can all laugh about it later when you've had some rest. Regardless, there is something that you should know. Today's commercial diapers are true wonders, the result of hours and hours of engineering and scientific diligence. I've even been told that they let "volunteer" toddlers in diapers filled with creamed corn loose on jungle gyms to monitor leakage. However, all this fantastic "superabsorbency" makes it virtually impossible to tell whether a newborn has wet his pants. Try tucking a small piece of tissue or some cotton balls onto the part of the diaper where your little one is most likely to aim a stream of urine (middle for girls, front for boys). This allows you to know with certainty whether or not Marge has successfully produced urine.

> ### EMERGENCY!
> Should you truly have concerns that your newborn is dehydrated, this is a medical emergency in the very young. A newborn who is difficult to wake to feed, has a sunken "soft spot" or dry mouth, or whose skin feels thick or doughy should be evaluated immediately by a medical professional.

*Bloody Diapers, Part 1: Did He Pee Blood?!* It is very rare for a newborn to actually have blood in his pee. If it is a girl, a small amount of bleeding from the vagina is completely normal. What is even more common is finding a pinkish orange staining of the diaper, in the area hit by urine. The uric acid found in urine can react with the material in the diaper and form pink crystals. It is absolutely not blood, is normal, and is 100 percent harmless. You don't need to change her diet or give it another thought. If you still truly believe there is blood in the urine, give your doctor a call, especially if the baby seems more irritable, is lethargic, or has a fever.

*Constipation/Diarrhea/Other Poop Issues.* Many a family, complete with Grandma, Grandpa, Aunt, Uncle, cousins, and neighbors, comes to the ER to report that the baby has not produced stool in two days, ten days, two hours, or [insert time period]. If you are lucky, maybe by the time you've waited six hours to see me, Billy will have laid a little present in his diaper, giving us all a hearty chuckle and you a quick trip back out the front door. However, more likely is that you will receive the following speech from me. All babies are different. Usually the first several stools are that thick, green, slimy product referred to as meconium. You don't really want to know what that is. Rather, you should just be thankful that after the first several stools, most babies begin producing something that resembles, well, um, creamed corn. However, some babies, especially those that are formula fed, will produce stools that look like anything from canned vegetables to normal adult formed stool. The consistency and color are of less interest to us than you might think. And some babies poop five times a day; some poop once a week. That is also not so exciting to me.

## WILL SHE EVER STOP?

Breastfed babies will usually poop several times a day in the first couple of weeks and by two months may have slowed down to weekly deposits. Soft poop is not constipated poop, no matter the frequency. Turning red, tensing the belly, grunting, and drawing up the legs are normal baby behavior, not a valid sign of constipation. You try pooping on your back with your butt clenched shut.

Constipation means that the stools are hard, rocklike, and difficult to pass. A baby is not necessarily "constipated" when he doesn't create stool on the expected time schedule laid out for him by anxious caregivers. In addition, all babies turn red and grunt and draw their legs up when they poop. It is rare that a newborn is actually constipated, and requires nothing more than a little patience and understanding.

If your baby produces *no* stool in the first seventy-two hours of life or if he produces rare stools that are very thin and ribbonlike, please call your pediatrician. In addition, an infant whose stools are completely white needs to be evaluated.

**Bloody Diapers, Part 2: Bloody Stools.** A very common cause of bloody poop in a newborn is swallowed maternal blood. In other words, he inadvertently took a swig on the way out. These stools are usually dark and tarry because the blood has passed all the way through the gut and been digested. If the blood is truly from the birthing experience, it should pass within the first couple of days of life.

Blood appears in the stool after the first couple of days most commonly under the following two conditions. Case one is that Billy is actually constipated and has passed a large, hard stool that is streaked with blood. This is the result of the large, difficult-to-pass stool creating tiny tears on its way out. These little rips in the skin are of little concern other than as a sign that the poops should be softer. If this is a one-time event, no worries, but if the stools are consistently very hard and large, talk to your pediatrician about appropriate ways to encourage softer poops in a tiny baby. More commonly in a newborn, the stool is loose, with strings of blood and mucus mixed throughout. This is truly bloody stool and someone should definitely hear about it. Most often the blood is the result of a condition called allergic colitis. When a baby becomes sensitive to something in his diet, the most common offending agents being cow's milk and soy proteins, the gut can become raw and inflamed and begin to bleed. Breastfed babies are not immune to allergic colitis since what Mom eats can show up in the milk. You should call your pediatrician, who can advise you on appropriate dietary changes, either for Mom or babe. Be aware that there may still be some blood in the stools for up to a couple of weeks while his gut heals.

Any newborn that is passing large amounts of blood, or anything that looks like pure blood or strawberry jelly, should be seen by his doctor. A baby who seems very irritable or lethargic, has fever, or has a tense or hard and distended belly should also be seen urgently. But remember that serious causes of bloody stools are quite rare in otherwise healthy newborn babies.

**King Arthur's Sword.** Circumcisions: There are arguments for and against what has become the most common elective surgical procedure in this country and should be discussed with your pediatrician prior to little Fred's arrival. Should you decide to circumcise your little football player, here are a few things you should know. There are a couple of common methods of circumcision in newborns and each comes with its own set of postprocedural care instructions. Follow your doctor's advice. However, what many physicians forget to warn new parents about is that healing circumcision wounds can look gross. When a wound heals in a warm, moist environment (as on a penis), it can look very white and goopy. This is normal and shouldn't panic you.

Once the wound has healed, the circumcised penis needs to be gently yet thoroughly cleaned at every diaper change with the remaining foreskin gently retracted to allow visualization and cleansing of the entire glans, or tip of the penis. Otherwise a buildup of smegma, which is just dead skin cells and looks like cottage cheese, can occur in the space between the foreskin and the glans. The other reason for gently retracting the foreskin during a diaper change is to prevent the development of adhesions, or scar tissue, between the remaining foreskin and glans, which can eventually make the foreskin no longer retractable. If this happens, the penis can look uncircumcised or it might actually become sucked into all that chubbiness on top of his pelvic bone and get stuck, like a magical disappearing penis trick. These conditions can be remedied, but in severe cases may require surgical correction. So maintain vigilance!

If you've elected to leave his little manlihood alone, then a diaper change is much simpler. The *uncircumcised* foreskin should never be forcibly retracted during cleansing of the penis. It will, with time, free itself from the glans and become retractable. Forceful retraction of a foreskin that is not yet ready to let go will cause pain, trauma, and possibly scar tissue and adhesions.

If you notice foul-smelling drainage or redness spreading or "streaking" (like paint streaks) up toward the belly following a circumcision, quickly alert your physician. In addition, an uncircumcised male may develop a condition where the foreskin becomes retracted and "stuck" behind the glans, looking like a little foreskin balloon hat on the glans. This is a medical emergency and warrants immediate attention.

***The Berries.*** A word about the newborn scrotum. Remember how those hormones are still coursing through his body? A full-term newborn boy will have a scrotum that is more adultlike in appearance. The testicles will hang low and the skin will be quite loose. As the hormones clear, the skin will tighten up and the scrotum will shrink in size and lay closer to the body. Therefore, in the first few weeks of life, it should be pretty easy to tell where the testicles are, confirm that there are indeed two of them, and that they are sitting where they should.

Sometimes the scrotum will appear uneven, with one side appearing fuller or more swollen than the other. The most common cause of swelling in the scrotum is called a hydrocele and is just a little collection of fluid. Other babies will have a hernia, which is created when pieces of bowel are able to slip down into the scrotum through an abnormal opening between the scrotum and the belly. Any worries should be directed to your pediatrician. If the swelling appears very painful, hard, or red, your doctor should hear about it right away.

*It's a Girl!* So as not to slight little Sally, let's give a few moments to the newborn vagina. Several days after birth you might find a small amount of blood coming from the vagina. All those hormones may have caused a little thickening of the lining of her uterus, which sheds as the hormone levels drop, similar to a little period. This in no way is considered a real period; it doesn't affect her development at puberty and is completely normal.

Let's say you find a firm little lump in the skin folds next to the vagina. This needs to be brought to the attention of your physician during regular business hours. It is possible to have an ovary migrate south. This definitely requires an evaluation by your doctor, both for planning surgical correction down the road as well as making sure there are no other (rare!) associated conditions.

## The Skin

*Blue Baby.* A slight bluish discoloration of the hands and feet and sometimes around the mouth (not inside the lips!) is called acrocyanosis and is normal. The heart is simply sending blood to the places that need it most. This may worsen in colder temperatures but is largely of no concern. Blue lips or tongues *do* need to be evaluated.

**ƎI I!**

A very pale, blue, or gray baby should be seen right away. If he does not seem to be breathing normally or seems floppy, sleepy, or unconscious, call 911. This is an emergency.

*Yellow Baby.* Some babies will develop a yellowish cast to their skin that we call jaundice. As a newborn poops, she clears out a substance called bilirubin. Bilirubin is produced by red blood cells and the liver and is normally cleared through the gut. The most common reason for a newborn to become jaundiced is an immature bilirubin-clearing system. If you think your little one is looking a bit yellow, check her eyes, because true jaundice will turn the whites of her eyes yellow. If her eyes remain sparkling white, but her skin still seems yellow, ask your pediatrician, but she's probably just got olive skin. In cases of true jaundice, your doctor may want to check her bilirubin level.

If the measured bilirubin is very high, special lights (a Bili-Blanket) or hospitalization may be necessary until the levels come down because extremely high bilirubin levels may affect a newborn's brain development. But for most babies, ensuring that she's pooping and drinking and careful observation are enough. Natural sunlight hastens the clearance of biliru-

**GUESSTIMATION**

The poor man's way of estimating the bilirubin level is seeing how far down on the body the yellow tinge travels. Yellowness that is confined to skin above the belly button is most likely within a safe range for a full-term baby, but we usually check the blood level just in case.

bin, so ask your doctor if a brief sit in front of the living room window is a good idea.

*Lacy Baby.* Some babies will have a very fine, lacy-looking appearance that typically worsens when cold. This is nothing to worry about. Put her pants on.

*Rashes.* Take a look at your baby's bum now because this is the last time it will look so healthy until she's in big-girl underpants. Diaper rash is a fact of life, but you've got at least a few days of peaceful diaper changes ahead. Keep everything as clean and as dry as possible, and when the spots appear, flip to the middle of the book.

As for other rashes in newborns, they are universal and rarely of interest. In the vast array of unsightly skin disorders that plague the newborn population, most can be labeled as either cradle cap or newborn crud. Newborn crud refers to the collection of skin afflictions appearing early in life, ranging from the perfectly harmless white bumps on the nose that we call milia to more severe and potentially dangerous rashes. Okay, that probably didn't make you feel too good. Just understand that babies are covered in all kinds of bumps and lumps and imperfections, and most are completely normal and nothing to worry about.

For example, pimples are pretty normal in wee ones. Newborn hormones rage like that of a teenager. After all, they were just living inside a virtual hormone factory for forty weeks. So, it should not come as any surprise that tiny little babies could have acne. Most clear up and require no treatment. Please try to resist the urge to pop her zits. Occasionally a little one will have more severe skin eruptions and may require some pharmaceutical intervention. See your pediatrician in this case.

As for cradle crap, um, cap, also known as seborrhea, this

is what we medical folks describe as a "greasy rash" (*mmm*) that often begins on the scalp and can course all the way down south to the toes. It's harmless but ugly. See "Rashes of the Scalp," on page 179 if your little one looks like she's getting a bit of dandruff.

When in doubt, ask your pediatrician.

*Stork Bites.* Flip the baby over and look at the back of his neck at the hairline. If there is a red "rash" or "spot" that feels like normal skin but is just strangely red, this is where the stork held the baby in his beak as he carried him through the sky on his way to your loving arms. Seriously, we call this a stork bite. This may go away by high school or it might be permanent. I still have mine.

*Angel Kisses.* Okay, flip him back over and look at his face. Do you see a spot similar to the stork bite on his forehead just over his eyes? If you do, you are very lucky because that is where the angels kissed him just before he left for earth. Again, laugh if you must, but we call this an angel kiss and it is more likely to disappear than the stork bite, although some will stick around. If it is really bothersome or refusing to fade and you are worried about his prom pictures, you can have it zapped with a laser down the road. No worries.

*Miscellaneous Spots and Dots.* There is something called a Mongolian spot, most commonly found on babies of darker-skinned ethnicities. This is just an area of abnormal pigmentation commonly found on the buttocks or lower spine. These can look like bruises but absolutely aren't; they are normal and nothing to worry about.

If you are being really vigilant about looking your new baby over, you might find a tiny red spot that disappears or pales significantly when pressed upon. That is a strawberry hemangioma. A hemangioma is a little abnormal blood vessel that continues to grow and grow over the first several months of life until it gradually recedes and fades away. Most of these are incredibly small, barely noticeable, and go away without making a fuss. However, some babies have rather large lesions, or lesions in areas such as over the eye or lip where a growing mass could cause problems and needs to be dealt with by a plastic surgeon or dermatologist. These little spots aren't usually visible immediately after birth, but kudos to you for your observance.

*Peeling Skin.* Yes, her skin is supposed to peel shortly after delivery. Leave it alone.

## Is She Supposed to Act This Way?

### Fun with Reflexes

Now for the entertainment section. Babies are born with all kinds of fantastically amusing reflexes that gradually disappear over the first several weeks of life. So gather your friends, strip down the baby, and get ready to have fun.

Two of the most basic newborn reflexes are simple rooting and grasping. If you place your finger in the palm of her hand, she will automatically grasp your finger. But you can do the same thing with her toes! And if you gently stroke her cheek, she will reflexively turn her head to that side. That is called rooting, and she is looking for food.

Now, stand her up and set her feet on the floor. She might lift her leg and look like she's walking. If you move her gently forward, you may be able to get two or three little steps out of her.

Next, flip her onto her belly and hold her up in the air with one hand, supporting her chest and belly. Gently run your finger down one side of her trunk and her whole body will curl up in that direction. Switch to the other side and she'll follow suit.

Finally, lay her on her back with her upper body a few inches off the floor in your hands. Suddenly drop your hands a few millimeters. Both arms should extend outward with open hands. This is called the startle reflex and is a good sign of an alert and intact brain.

Well, folks, that's all the time we have for fun with reflexes. Now when you inadvertently make any of the above movements that elicit a reflex, you'll know what you've done and you'll know that she's doing just what a newborn is supposed to do. If you're now worried that your kid is missing a reflex or isn't performing them properly, do not panic. Wait until regular office hours and ask your pediatrician to take a look. It's most likely your technique and nothing more.

## Shakes, Twitches, and Jerks

All babies, especially newborns, twitch and jerk about to a certain extent. Sometimes it is more apparent when she is on the cusp of a lovely slumber. This is almost always normal. If you are in any way worried about her movements, try to capture them on video and take the clip to your doctor's office. If a newborn does seem to be having rhythmic jerking, particularly of one side of the body or the whole body, that is lasting for more than a couple of beats, you need to call your pediatrician immediately.

## The Baby Sleeps Too Much/Too Little

The amount of time newborns sleep varies wildly between babies. On average, they sleep about sixteen hours a day. But this is just an *average*, which means that some infants may seem to never sleep and others need to be wrapped in wet towels before they will eat. What is more important than the actual amount of time the baby sleeps is paying attention to what kind of baby *you've* got. If you have a baby who seems to be awake every hour but suddenly you are having trouble waking her up, I'd be concerned and want her checked out. Conversely, if you have to strip that little kid naked and place cold rags on her back to get her to latch on, but suddenly she's screaming and inconsolable for an extended period of time, I'd also want to see that baby.

And in the end, whether you have a baby who sleeps 23.5 hours a day or one who sleeps 3, he's sleeping on his back. Period. Since the Back to Sleep campaign was launched by the AAP in 1992, death from SIDS (sudden infant death syndrome) has dropped significantly, by some counts as much as 30 to 50 percent. So I don't care if he seems to sleep better on his tummy or if Grandma thinks he's going to choke on his spit. Put him on his back. He'll get used to it. He's not going to choke or have trouble breathing. Yes, his head might get a little flat in the back but not if you give him enough "tummy time" when he's awake.

## What about Feeding It?

### Breastfeeding Issues

Newborns: Let's just lay it on the line. Breastfeeding is best. Besides all that lovey-dovey stuff about bonding and feeling close to your baby, human breast milk is the perfect food for human babies. Just like cow's milk is the perfect food for baby cows. Not only is it designed to provide little humans with all the nutrients they need, it is perfectly digestible by the little human. On top of that, the health benefits are undeniable. Breastfed infants have fewer ear infections, fewer respiratory infections, just plain fewer infections. They have fewer allergies. Some people even claim breastfed infants have higher IQs. And there are benefits for Mom, including reducing the risk of certain types of breast and ovarian cancers. Plus you can zip your old pants up sooner. And the list goes on. But as great as breastfeeding is, sometimes it can be hard to get started and sometimes it just doesn't work at all.

## WHAT THE EXPERTS SAY

The official recommendation of the American Academy of Pediatrics is exclusive breastfeeding for the first six months of life followed by the continuation of breastfeeding until at least one year of life and as long as mutually desired. Newborns should be nursed approximately eight to twelve times every twenty-four hours until full (around ten to fifteen minutes) and at the first signs of interest, such as increased alertness or rooting. Newborns should be awakened to feed if four hours have passed since their last snack.

How many infants do I see in the ER for breastfeeding problems? More than you might believe. It is amazing to me that families are sent home from the hospital before Mom has mastered the art of waking up a sleeping baby and getting it to put a large nipple in its mouth and before the kid figures out how to get himself a snack. Breastfeeding is more work for a baby than a bottle and nipple. Rather than simply sucking, he has to pull his tongue forward and "milk" (pun intended) the fluid from the breast. That is why putting just the nipple in the baby's mouth won't get you anywhere. Good breastfeeding technique demands that the baby get as much of the areola into his mouth as possible. It's tiring, so if you have a lazy baby, you're going to have to do a little encouraging. After all, any baby can let milk passively fall into his mouth from a rubber nipple. So if it means stripping him naked, pinching his toes, and prying open his mouth, then that's what it is going to take.

Your breast is empty in about fifteen to twenty minutes, so any sucking that goes on beyond that time is simply recreational. Babies spend two to three hours a day on "nonnutritive" sucking. It's one of those developmental things. That's what thumbs and pacifiers are for. Not your cracked and bleeding nipples. But, you say, he's so hungry, he's growing, he needs more milk. Your breasts produce milk on a *frequency* basis, not on a duration of sucking session basis. So to make more milk, feed more often. Eventually your breasts will increase their production to meet Buddy's big appetite and you can space your feedings back out a bit.

There are circumstances in which breastfeeding is simply not possible. That's okay. Your kid is still going to grow up big and strong and will sneak out at night and steal the car and that has absolutely nothing to do with whether or not he got

### A Word about Water

All the water a baby needs is in his daily formula or breast milk intake. Adding up to 1 ounce a day of water is perfectly safe albeit unnecessary. Beware that little baby kidneys just haven't yet finessed the difficult task of balancing waters and salts. Therefore, a baby who is given larger amounts of water or whose formula is watered down (a dangerous technique employed by some parents who are trying to make formula last longer out of economical concerns) may result in very low blood sodium. If low enough, baby can have seizures and possible brain injury.

the dreaded *commercial formula!* However, allow me to let you in on a little secret. Infant formulas must adhere to a pretty strict set of government rules with regard to content and vitamins and all that jazz. So essentially, the expensive brand names and the generic versions are exactly the same. Maybe they tweak a little of this or that, but you will not poison your child if you buy plain old generic Safeway formula. And with the money you save, you can pay the bail after Buddy steals the car and gets arrested.

## The Baby Eats Too Much/Too Little

Whether you are bottle feeding or breastfeeding, how do you know if he's getting enough? Certainly there is someone who is trying to convince you that he needs more. I'm truly shocked on occasion by some families who come to the ER complaining that their infant is vomiting only to find out that this two-week-old is being fed an eight-ounce bottle every three hours. Honestly! The poor little guy. I'd throw up too if I had to drink a gallon of milk every couple of hours.

On the first day of life a newborn's stomach is about the size of a marble and can hold only a tiny amount of fluid. His stomach capacity increases gradually over the first few days until he's taking in a good amount of milk. On average, a newborn drinks between twelve and twenty-four ounces of formula or breast milk in a twenty-four-hour period. As long as he's pooping and peeing and gaining weight, that's the amount that is right for him. As for frequency, remember that breast milk is perfectly designed for little ones, so these babies are going to eat more frequently, perhaps every one-and-a-half to two hours. Formula is more difficult for a baby to digest than breast milk and thus tends to stick around a little longer, so most bottle-fed infants will eat every three to four hours.

## INTRODUCING SOLIDS

There is no room for solids in a newborn's diet. None. You may see these "infant feeders" that are designed to shovel solid food into the back of an infant's throat. This is unnecessary from a nutritional standpoint. And potentially harmful, as a newborn is not physically mature enough to handle solid foods properly and the early introduction of solids has been associated with the development of food allergies.

## Not Gaining Weight

How much weight should she be gaining? Most newborns will lose up to 10 percent of their body weight in the first several days after birth. By two weeks of age, she should have regained all that lost weight and possibly more. A newborn who is growing as expected should be gaining a half to one full ounce a day, which translates to a pound every one to two weeks. If you have any concerns that she is not gaining weight appropriately, don't wait—call your pediatrician immediately.

# the ABCs

## Airway, Breathing, and Circulation

Remember "Airway, Breathing, and Circulation"? The "ABCs" of resuscitation? If you've taken your CPR class, this phrase should be beaten into you. Even medical professionals who resuscitate people every day know that when something changes or a patient worsens in any way, it's best to go right back to the beginning and the ABCs. Anyway, just as you were perplexed and worried by the strange noises and funny breathing patterns made by your newborn, as your child grows, the noises and worries continue. Same goes for every skipped heartbeat or cry of chest pain. Remember that most things are normal and not a problem.

## CPR

Seriously, if you've taken a CPR course, good for you! But *beware*. Recently the American Heart Association began endorsing "compression-only CPR" for adults, meaning no mouth-to-mouth. This is *not* a good idea for children. Kids don't have heart attacks. Their hearts stop because they aren't breathing. In little ones, resuscitation is all about oxygen.

## Airway and Breathing

### Respiratory Distress

There is a difference between a child who is wheezing but laughing, drinking, and playing (the "Happy Wheezer") and a kid who is actually working to breathe. Babies and little kids can't tell you when they are having trouble breathing, but maintaining good air exchange and appropriate oxygen levels is vitally important for their heart, brain, and other organs. Signs that a child is having more trouble breathing and needs attention include coughing, breathing hard or fast, or in very severe and far-gone cases, too slowly. The nostrils of a little baby may move in and out (flaring) or they may bob their heads up and down. Babies and children who are in distress may make a "grunting" noise with every breath. Kids will use all of their muscles to get in enough air, so look for pulling of the skin between the ribs, over the collarbone, or under the rib cage (retractions). A child who is verbal but can't say a full sentence without pausing to breathe needs attention, as does a baby or toddler who looks like breathing has become work. If your baby is smiling and drinking and interacting and is playful, you're okay. But the minute breathing changes from an instinct to a job, call your doctor right away.

### Cough

My mother says she used to lie awake at night, listening to me hack and cough and cough and hack. Even now, if I so much as clear my throat, I get a nasty look. All babies cough and sneeze. Coughing and sneezing are reflexes that occur when the little hairs (called cilia) lining your airways get irritated. So if a little dust finds its way into your lungs, it sticks on to your cilia, which annoys them, and then you cough. Anything that irritates your airways may cause coughing. Dust, food, snot from a cold, a stray earring back, and so on. Most coughing in infants is due to a cold or other infection. If the cough is due to something in the *upper airway* (the nose or throat), it should be pretty loose, although it can sound mighty junky. The cough usually gets worse at night too, because all that snot rolls down the back of the throat and triggers a coughing spell. Lots of parents say they can "feel" the cough in the chest and are sure that there is something more serious going on, like the dreaded pneumonia. However, in babies and little kids, a simple cold can cause enough mucus in the nose and big airways of the lungs to rattle around and make lots of noise and vibration. Some kids (and grown-ups!) may cough hard enough to make them throw up, or develop small bruises (called petechiae) on the face and neck. If your baby has a cold and is coughing to the point of puking, he may have bronchiolitis or another infection, such as pertussis (whooping cough). Bronchiolitis is an infection that occurs only in children less than two years of age. For kids with a family history of asthma, or those who are older than the typical age for bronchiolitis, I would be mighty suspicious that a child who is coughing so violently may actually be wheezing. Forceful coughing may also cause a little bruising of the whites of the eyes, which looks like bright red spots on the eyeball. All of this may look scary, but is honestly perfectly normal.

As difficult as it is to listen to your little one gasp and snort and cough her way through yet another cold, it is so much more difficult to believe that there isn't something more you can be doing. Alas, cough and cold medicines just don't work that well for us, and not at all for babies and children.

## RED SPOTS

Tiny broken blood vessels look like little red spots and are called petechiae. Such a rash on the face and neck can occur due to coughing or vomiting forcefully. However, if the rash exists below the neck, it might be caused by an infection, not just straining, and your doctor needs to know right away.

Unfortunately, there have been serious side effects and even deaths associated with their usage. In 2007, the FDA issued a public health advisory recommending against the use of cough and cold medicine in children, particularly those less than two years of age. A recent study suggested that around 7,000 children are sent to ERs every *year* because of these drugs. As a result, most "infant" preparations of over-the-counter cough and cold medicines have been removed from the store shelves. Yes, it is true that most of these cases were the result of inappropriate usage or dosing of these medicines. However, since they don't work, and even at "recommended" doses may have significant side effects (such as sleepiness or crying and irritability), most physicians advise against giving them to chil-

## BEES DON'T COUGH

Research suggests that a spoonful of honey at bedtime provides better cough relief (and better sleep!) in kids than either traditional cough medicine or no treatment. Go ahead and try it, but remember that honey is recommended *only* for kids over the age of one, since younger babies might be susceptible to a certain type of infection, called botulism, that can result from ingesting honey or corn syrup.

dren. Pain and fever relief, lots of fluids, saline nose drops, and mindless television (or a good book) are really all we can suggest.

## Croup

While most coughing is of the normal old cold type, there are certain types of cough or airway "noise" that are specific to certain infections. Croup is a viral infection that causes swelling of the area below the vocal cords. Classically, a kid has a cold for a couple of days and then wakes suddenly in the middle of the night barking like a circus seal. Some kids make a terrible whooping noise every time they breathe in. The kid can look terrible and as if she is just struggling to breathe. So in a panic, Mom and Dad run out the door in slippers and robe, heading for the nearest hospital. But by the time they arrive, the little walrus has disappeared and the kid looks pretty okay. This is croup. In you or me, when we get a virus that causes swelling around our vocal cords, we lose our voice, which most people call laryngitis. The airway of a baby or young child is shaped differently and the swelling happens below the vocal cords, where the little kid airway is the most narrow. This causes the classic "barky" cough and may cause something called stridor, which is a harsh noise made when breathing inward.

A change in temperature seems to relieve some kids, which is why rushing out into the cold night air on the way to the hospital seems to help. Although the steamy mist we give in the hospital was proven to be useless, some people still believe that steam might help. It's worth a try if your wee one wakes at 2 a.m. barking like a dog. Just run the hot water in the bathroom to make a steam bath. On the other hand, you can also try opening the freezer door and seeing if the cold air helps. If you are worried about wasting electricity, stick her out on the porch. The sensation of not being able to pull air in properly is probably pretty upsetting, but crying only makes the symptoms worse, so try to calm yourself and find a way to soothe and distract your little one. Most of the time, simply holding your child and calming him down will help ease the coughing and noise. In fact, that is probably what the change in temperature is doing. If your kid looks and feels better after a bit, you can go back to sleep and call your pediatrician in the morning. However, if your baby seems to be really struggling to breathe, especially when he is calm and not crying, is making a lot of noise, using extra muscles around the neck and chest to breathe, or is turning blue, he needs to be seen immediately. And if you are unsure, call your pediatrician.

## ON THE WAY IN

If your doctor decides your child needs to go to the ER but is not sick enough to require an ambulance, try cranking down the car windows if it is winter, or cranking up the AC in the summer. The cold air might ease her coughing.

If you have to go to the emergency room, the most common treatment is a medicine either by mouth or by shot that will help calm the swelling in the airway. The medicine doesn't work for several hours, but most kids with croup get a little worse before they get better, so the medicine may prevent another episode later that day or the next night. If a child is making a lot of noise or struggling to breathe, an aerosol treatment of epinephrine may be given, which should immediately reduce the swelling. The only stinker about the aerosol is that once it's given, a kid usually needs to stay in the ER for two to four hours to make sure the really severe symptoms don't return. Inconvenient as it may be, you really do want to be in the ER if your child suddenly develops more trouble breathing. If a kid needs more than one aerosol treatment, we will often admit her to the hospital to be watched very closely. Fortunately, most kids do just fine at home, spreading the virus to all their little buddies in the neighborhood.

## Bronchiolitis

Parents always confuse the following two words: *bronchitis* and *bronchiolitis*. Bronchitis is an inflammation of the larger airways and does not occur in children. Bronchiolitis is a disease that *only* little kids (under age two) get. *Bronchiolitis* refers to a viral inflammation and swelling of the smaller airways of the lungs, the bronchioles. Bronchiolitis usually occurs in the late fall and winter months and is characterized by a few days of a cold followed by a gradually worsening cough, faster-than-normal breathing, and wheezing. Several different viruses may cause bronchiolitis, although the most

## IS YOUR KID A SMOKER?

**Myth 1:** A kid can have bronchitis. **Fact:** Bronchitis is a disease that old people and smokers get. Children do not.

**Myth 2:** Bronchitis is treated with antibiotics. **Fact:** Antibiotics have been shown to be useless for the treatment of bronchitis, probably since most cases are viral.

well known is the respiratory syncytial virus, or RSV. The vast majority of babies weather through just fine and get better within several days, although the cough may last for several weeks. Unfortunately, you can get RSV more than once. So if Freddy had it as a baby, don't think he can't get it ten more times and pass it on to every new sibling you bring home for him.

Bronchiolitis can be a serious illness in some babies. Newborns, for instance, may rarely "forget" to breathe when infected with RSV. Once a baby is older than one or two months of age, this phenomenon ends, but is important to remember if your baby is around smaller infants who may be more vulnerable. What is more, infants who are born prematurely, have heart or lung problems, and certain other conditions may tend to have a much more severe course of illness and should be watched closely.

The vast majority of babies with bronchiolitis, as I've said, do just fine, other than having a nasty cough that lingers (more than two to four weeks). However, some babies will develop severe trouble breathing and may need oxygen or even (rarely!) to be put on a ventilator, or breathing machine, to help them get through the worst of it. These babies clearly need to be in the hospital. Most babies are going to drink or eat less than normal because they don't feel well. However, a few babies may find themselves breathing so fast that they can't feed properly or are stopping to cough and choke while drinking and run the risk of becoming dehydrated. These infants may need to receive IV fluids or stay in the hospital a few days.

The worst part about bronchiolitis is that there is really *nothing we can do*. Some doctors will try certain asthma medications, especially if a lot of people in the family have asthma, but all the evidence we have suggests this is likely a waste of time for most babies. Babies who have bouts of wheezing all winter, or with every new cold, may be at higher risk for developing asthma or may have another problem, such as reflux, so it might be worth mentioning this to your doctor. But regular old bronchiolitis is really just a waiting game. As long as your baby can drink enough to stay hydrated and isn't working so hard to breathe that it looks like breathing has become her full-time job, there is nothing to do. No cough medicines. No magic solution. Sorry.

## Pneumonia

I used to tell people I had "ammonia" when I was a little kid, but since I wasn't cleaning the toilets, they usually understood that I meant "pneumonia." Pneumonia is an infection that settles *in* the lungs, usually in one part of the lung (a lobe). Kids with pneumonia may have a cough and breathe faster than normal, even when their fever comes down. Some kids with pneumonia will have vomiting as their only symptom, and older kids may complain of belly pain. Sometimes a doctor can hear the infection in part of the lung with a stethoscope, and other times you can't hear a thing. Pneumonia is tricky like that.

Both bacterial *and* viral infections can cause pneumonia,

### THE DREADED PNEUMONIA

Pneumonia is simply an infection that has settled in the lungs. Viruses are responsible for the majority of pneumonias in young children, which means antibiotics will often be ineffective.

which is important to understand because antibiotics *only* treat infections caused by bacteria. They do *nothing* for viral infections. Unfortunately, it can be very difficult to know whether a patient with pneumonia has a bacterial or a viral infection. The decision to give antibiotics to a patient is based on many different things and is a very imprecise science. The reassuring thing about pneumonia in kids is that the vast majority will have a viral, rather than a bacterial, infection. So most kids weather through just fine with nothing more than a little love and tenderness.

Another problem with "pneumonia" is that it is very often overdiagnosed. The sad part about my "ammonia" story is that I actually had uncontrolled, unrecognized asthma. I was coughing and coughing with every cold, but because I had a cough and a fever, I was given antibiotics for my "pneumonia," rather than treated for my asthma. But this was two hundred years ago, when I was a little girl, and we just didn't know as much about asthma in kids as we do now. What we *do* know now is that kids shouldn't get pneumonia more than once. A kid with a history of "pneumonia" three times has probably been misdiagnosed.

## RERUNS

An otherwise healthy child will not have repeated episodes of pneumonia. It's probably undiagnosed and undertreated *asthma*, which some people refer to as reactive airway disease, because no one likes to label a kid with a word that sounds so depressing. But don't be afraid of a diagnosis of asthma, because once you have the right diagnosis, your kid can get the right treatment!

Because pneumonia can mimic so many other illnesses and vice versa, most of us consider pneumonia to be a diagnosis we make "clinically," not based just on a chest X-ray. Chest X-rays to look for pneumonia may be falsely normal, especially early in the illness. Or they may show areas of the lung that are abnormal, but can't help us decide if the abnormality is because of infection or something else, such as asthma. So insisting on a chest X-ray for your child is not really beneficial. There are times when an X-ray is helpful, but your doctor can make this decision based on your child's appearance, how long he's been sick, and a host of other factors.

Kids who are having trouble breathing, breathing very hard or fast, using extra muscles, and acting like breathing is work probably need to be seen right away and possibly kept in the hospital. Some babies and children with pneumonia will need oxygen, so they need to stay in the hospital too. And for those little ones who decide vomiting is their symptom of choice, a few may need to get IV fluids, either in the ER or as a patient in the hospital. Some kids might need their antibiotics through an IV too, not because the antibiotics work any better this way, but because they are throwing up too much to hold down their medicine.

The most important thing for a parent to know is that if you feel your kid is acting more ill, or breathing harder or faster, especially when her fever is back to normal, don't hesitate to call your doctor.

## Wheezing and Asthma

A child who coughs until he throws up is, in my book, wheezing until proven otherwise. Wheezing happens when the muscles around the tiny airways in the lungs become very twitchy and begin to spasm. This makes the airways even narrower and it is difficult for air to flow out of the lungs. When we listen with a stethoscope, we hear high-pitched noises in the lungs when the patient breathes. If the lungs are very full of air and little air is flowing outward, it may be very difficult to hear anything.

The reason it is important to know if your child is wheezing is not just because this may be a sign that she has asthma or another illness, but also because it is something that we can actually do something about! Not every kid who wheezes will develop asthma. Some children wheeze with every cold, which is considered a mild form of asthma, and grow out of it later. If a child does have asthma, which really just means repeated episodes of wheezing, it is important that she be appropriately diagnosed, so that episodes can be both treated and prevented. A history of repeated episodes of "pneumonia," a history of allergies or a family member with allergies or asthma, coughing to the point of vomiting, or severe coughing or fast breathing with every cold are all big clues that a child may have asthma.

If your child already has a diagnosis of asthma (or reactive airway disease, same thing) and you feel his symptoms are worsening, call your doctor without hesitation. Early interruption of an asthma exacerbation may mean the difference between a night of coughing and a week in the intensive care unit.

As always, if your baby seems to be working to breathe, is using extra muscles in her ribs and belly to breathe, or is making a grunting noise with every breath, she needs to be seen immediately. Older children who are unable to speak a full sentence are in significant distress as well and need urgent attention.

## Noisy Breathing

Think back to high school physics. Do you remember Poiseuille's law? I'll refresh you. As air flows through a tube, it becomes more and more turbulent the smaller the tube. Translation: Little tiny noses sound really noisy when air goes through them. Now add a tiny little booger and the noise increases exponentially. It's like a truck going through a wind tunnel. To quote one of my dear pediatrician friends: "I swear, Lara, I lie in bed unable to sleep because my kid is in the next room, making so much noise, he sounds like a pig in s*$%!" If your baby turns out to be a noisy breather, you are not alone. All babies squirm and sputter to some extent. A few babies actually have a floppy airway and are exceptionally noisy breathers, especially when lying on their back. Most babies outgrow this and it is no problem. Remember that newborns and small infants are *obligate nose breathers*, which means that they *have* to breathe through the nose. They can't sleep with their mouth hanging wide open and flies going in and out. That is what makes them so cute. But it also means that they are going to be noisy little critters. Again, as long as it seems to bother only you, and she is able to suck and feed and sleep without effort, it's fine. Using a bulb syringe might help to clear out some of the mucus, or a bit of saline drops can help thin the snot. If you are very concerned, mention it to your pediatrician. In very severe cases, some babies with floppy airways need a specialist to evaluate them and make sure there are no other reasons for the floppy airway, but this is very, very rare.

## Not Breathing

By now your little one should have grown out of that silly practice of "periodic breathing." Go back to Chapter 1 if you've already forgotten. Anyway, as an infant gets older, she may still have times where she holds her breath or appears not to be breathing. As long as the pauses are only a few seconds long, the baby *never changes color*, and begins breathing again with no help from you, this is normal. A baby who stops breathing for *any* period of time that includes a change in color or level of consciousness needs to be seen right away. In older babies (older than six months) and toddlers, true episodes of not breathing, called apnea, are extremely rare and are more likely conscious episodes of breath holding. The child should be awake and alert.

> **911!**
>
> A baby who turns blue inside (not around!) the lips or tongue, or appears limp or unconscious during a pause in breathing, needs to be seen *immediately* and you should call 911. A baby who is forgetting to breathe will often start again with stimulation, such as flicking the feet or rubbing firmly on the breastbone. This should hold you until the ambulance arrives.

And this brings us to a quirky toddler behavior that can begin in late infancy and continue on until preschool. Some toddlers (very rude and thoughtless, I think) have breath-holding spells. This is when a kiddo (usually) begins to cry (or is just startled or upset) and then suddenly holds his breath, turns blue, and passes out. Then he might twitch a few muscles for a couple of seconds, begin breathing, and wake up. As if nothing had happened. This is most disturbing for a parent. The key to diagnosing a breath-holding spell is that the event universally follows some emotional response to a stimulus, either a sudden startle when another kid grabs his toy, or a bloodcurdling scream when she doesn't get her way. While upsetting, it is important to remember that the little angel isn't consciously making herself pass out. That said, many toddlers will learn that a breath-holding spell can get them what they want, and little Claire may hold her parents prisoner with the threat of crying. One must not give in. She doesn't need a cookie every time she wants one. Be strong. She *will* outgrow this and she will *not* give herself brain damage. Those few seconds without oxygen are not long enough to cause her any harm, unless she gets too fat from eating so many cookies.

## Choking

They are noisy little critters. A baby who appears to gag and "choke" and blow bubbles is probably just doing her baby thing. A normal baby with a normal brain should be able to protect her own airway from spit and milk and anything else that tries to hit her own lungs. She does this by gagging and closing off her vocal cords so that nothing can slip by. As long as she turns red or reddish purple (never blue or very pale), is awake and struggling, and recovers by herself, she's just doing her job. Praise her, don't panic.

A baby who truly does choke on something, be it food or a forgotten Lego piece, is keeping her own airway open if she is coughing and making noise. If she appears to be in any distress, call 911 immediately. A child who is choking and

> ⊖ | | !
> Any baby who is truly choking and making no noise, or who is turning blue, needs immediate attention. Call 911.

## HOT DOGS AREN'T THE ONLY NO-NO

Babies and little kids are great at biting, but not so good at chewing. Firm, round foods should always be thoroughly chopped. Hot dogs should be peeled, sliced lengthwise, and chopped into little pieces, never served sliced only across. If it looks like it can plug up his airway, it can. Some foods that are particularly dangerous for kids under age four (or those who gulp without chewing) include: hot dogs, popcorn, whole grapes, seeds and nuts, chewing gum, hard candy, and anything that is a "chunk," like pieces of apple, carrot, meat, and cheese. Very sticky or gooey items are also high risk, like peanut butter and taffy.

suddenly stops struggling or appears limp or unconscious needs immediate attention. If the choking episode has passed on its own, and she seems fine, without further episodes of coughing or gagging, and is able to drink and eat normally, you can certainly give your pediatrician a call to let her know what happened, but it sounds like everything is fine.

## CHOKING PREVENTION

Little ones explore the world with all of their senses, including their mouths. Be mindful of everything that is within young Julia's reach, making sure that small toys (or parts), batteries, coins, marbles, pen caps, and the like are securely stowed. Latex balloons may look pretty, but pose a serious threat to a youngster (even up to school age!) who chooses to bite, pop, and inhale. This is also why I'm going to get mad if you try to entertain your kid by blowing up my exam gloves.

## Pertussis (Whooping Cough)

I was once seeing a baby in the emergency room for a "cough," and as soon as I had introduced myself, the dad launched into a story of how he had a cough for several weeks that was pretty bad, but then the baby got a cold and after several days starting coughing and coughing, to the point of throwing up! And what was really weird was how she made this "Whoop!" at the end of every coughing fit. That, my friends, is the classic story for pertussis, or whooping cough.

Pertussis is a bacterial infection that initially causes symptoms similar to a regular cold, but after one to two weeks a severe cough develops that can lead to vomiting and even bruising of the face and whites of the eyes. Pertussis is known as whooping cough because a patient will literally "Whoop!" at the end of a coughing jag. Not everyone will do so, however, with many babies and children simply coughing to the point of vomiting. Everyone forgot about pertussis for a while, when kids began receiving routine immunizations against the disease. We've now learned that the immunization is not perfect and can wear off, meaning that we still see quite a few cases every year. This does *not*, however, mean you shouldn't immunize your child against pertussis! The more people who aren't immunized in a community, the more likely it is that an infection can flourish and cause illness in both the immunized *and* the unimmunized. Pertussis causes an uncomfortable and annoying illness in older kids and adults, but can be extremely serious, even fatal, in babies.

If your doctor is concerned about pertussis, a lab test can confirm the diagnosis, but the results are not immediate, so antibiotics may be started while waiting for the test results. Antibiotics will lessen both the recovery time and the severity of symptoms, but your child won't get immediately better and the illness will still run its course. Treatment will prevent him from giving it to other children and adults. Babies under one year, and especially those younger than six months, may be admitted to the hospital while establishing the diagnosis because the smaller the baby, the more likely he is to become severely ill.

## The Heart and the Circulatory System

### Turning Blue

Just like in newborns, a slight bluish discoloration of the hands and feet and sometimes around the mouth (not the actual lips!) is called acrocyanosis and is normal. The blueness around the mouth may be pretty noticeable in very pale kids and may come and go. The heart is simply sending blood to the places that need it most. This may worsen in colder temperatures but is largely of no concern. However, you should mention this to your pediatrician, especially if it happens frequently or when he is all warm and toasty.

Should the lips or tongue ever turn blue, or the baby in general seems to have a paler, blue, or gray appearance to his skin, he needs to be evaluated. If he seems alert and is breathing, call your pediatrician. The reasons for a bluish appear-

### 911!

If a baby ever appears blue, very pale, or grayish and does not seem to be breathing normally or seems floppy, sleepy, or unconscious, call 911. This is an emergency.

ance are vast, ranging from certain home-cooked vegetables to heart problems. Most babies who have a brief "blue spell" and return to normal have just experienced a small choking episode or have heartburn. But every baby who turns blue needs to be seen immediately.

## Chest Pain

In adults, a complaint of "chest pain" probably gets you prompt admission to the emergency room, with all kinds of testing before the doctor even sees you. In an otherwise healthy kid, however, "chest pain" will probably get you four hours in the corner of the waiting room, watching old Jerry Springer reruns and eating vending machine Cheese Whiz on a cracker. The fact is that chest pain in children is very rarely related in any way to the heart. Chest pain in kids is most commonly pain in the muscles and cartilage of the chest wall, which can occur after vigorous play, coughing, and the like. Pushing along the front ribs and the chest bone, or sternum, causes the exact same pain as that which the child complained about.

Other causes of chest pain in children can be asthma or pneumonia, which are generally accompanied by a cough and possibly fever. A painful rash, such as shingles or poison ivy, could cause pain, so be sure to take a peek under his shirt. Heartburn can certainly cause chest pain in kids. And a few true heart conditions, such as an abnormally fast rhythm, may also cause chest pain, although *cardiac* causes of chest pain in kids are extremely rare. If your child is complaining of chest pain and appears otherwise alert and awake and is not having trouble breathing (other than crying that it hurts), have her rest for a bit and try a dose of pain medicine, such as ibuprofen. If, however, she appears extremely uncomfortable, is having more trouble breathing, is very pale, or is otherwise unwell, call your doctor.

## Murmurs

Now you are panicked, because you just got back from a checkup at the doctor's office and someone has heard a "murmur." So you've run straight here to see if you should panic. The answer is *no*. A murmur is heard with a stethoscope and is nothing more than the sound of blood rushing through the heart and blood vessels. In a normal adult heart, you wouldn't expect to hear a murmur because the blood would be smoothly running over normal muscles and heart valves, hidden deep under thick layers of skin, muscle, fat, and bone. However, little kids have a lot less body between a stethoscope and their hearts. In perfectly healthy babies and small kids, murmurs are quite common and often totally normal. In a thin preschooler, it is very common to hear a musical type of murmur that is entirely normal. In kids with fever, the normal increase in heart rate may make the blood flow a bit faster, creating a murmur. In tiny babies, the blood vessels bringing blood into the lungs may be very tiny and we can hear a murmur in the back and armpits. So, hearing a "murmur" is not necessarily anything bad.

### GOOD EARS

My cardiology friends say that a good cardiologist can hear a murmur in every newborn and all preschoolers. Some folks say that all kids will have a murmur at some time in their lives. No need to panic!

On the other hand, some murmurs will be caused by an abnormality of the structure of the heart, such as a hole between the big pumping chambers. Some of these anomalies will fix themselves with time and some won't and will require medication or even surgery. And this is why we listen for a murmur every time we use our stethoscope. Because of all the murmurs we hear, a small number will require evaluation by a cardiologist, or heart specialist, and we want to be sure that we don't miss something as important as a problem with a baby's heart. If your pediatrician decides to send your infant to a cardiologist, she still may be absolutely fine. Your doctor just wants an expert in murmurs to listen and decide whether any further testing needs to be done. So don't freak out if your kid gets a referral to a heart doctor.

## Beats and Rhythm

How fast should your baby's heart be beating? The heart of a fetus will usually beat at about 120 to 140 beats per minute. That is pretty fast, considering that your heart rate is about 70, except when you are reading this book and it jumps up to 100. After birth, a newborn's heart may beat between 80 and 180 beats per minute. Over the first year of life, the maximum normal heart rate slows down a bit, and most of us consider a heart rate of 80 to 100 to be quite normal in a one-year-old. From there the range of normal heart rates decreases over time, until about the age of ten, when the adult rate of 50 to 90 beats per minute is considered normal. Crying, fever, pain, and dehydration are just a few of the reasons that a heart rate may be higher than normal. A lower-than-normal heart rate is less common and may be more worrisome, indicating a problem with either a baby's oxygen levels or the heart's electrical system.

When do you panic? Well, I don't know why you'd want to take your kid's pulse, but if you get it in your head to try, a very fast heartbeat that is "too fast to count" and doesn't come down when she stops struggling to get away from you should prompt a call to your doctor. But really, you should leave the counting of a heart rate to the professionals. Even we sometimes find it tough in a wiggly baby. More important, if your baby seems to be having trouble breathing, is having to pause during feedings to catch her breath, or turns blue, she needs to be seen right away.

In young children, a slight irregularity of the heart rate can occur with breathing. This is called sinus arrhythmia and is the response of the heart's own speed sensors to the changes in pressure within the chest that occur with breathing. In school-age kids, this change may be very pronounced, sending more than one kid my way with a note from the school nurse about an "irregular heartbeat." If you are, for whatever reason, feeling your child's heartbeat and notice that it seems to be speeding up and slowing down, don't panic. If she's old enough, have her hold her breath. This should make the heart rate stay about the same speed and tell you that everything is normal.

# the noggin and nervous system

This chapter is *not* meant to give you new reasons to worry. Problems with a baby's brain and nervous system, the bones of the skull, or the size and shape of the head are really rare. Even a serious head injury from a good whack to the noggin is pretty rare. Your pediatrician will be routinely monitoring the growth of your child's head, the size of the soft spot, and her strength and development. Your job as a parent is *not* to obsess about these little things. Rather, if you have any concerns, raise them with your doctor and let her do the worrying for you. That said, I'll cover a few of the basic normal and not-so-normal things that concern parents when it comes to their kid's brain, including a few of those weird baby and toddler behaviors that can be funny and scary at the same time.

## The Skull and Brain

### Head Injuries

So she's hit her head. Or her brother took a bat to it. Either way, know that kids' heads are pretty hard. Essentially *any* blow to the head can be called a head injury. Decisions about the seriousness of the injury are based on several criteria. Believe me when I say that we see many, many head injuries a day. And the vast majority of kids are absolutely fine. If she is crying and alert, you can take a breath and read the rest of this section.

## 911!

If your child has hit her head and is unconscious or having a seizure, call 911.

The younger the baby, the more likely it is that your pediatrician would like to hear about a head injury. Babies have these wonderful soft spots that act as "pop-off" valves in case of injury to the brain. In the rare instance that the baby did sustain some bruising or bleeding inside her head, these pop-off valves will allow some pressure and swelling around the brain to occur without her developing the more typical signs of a head injury, such as confusion and vomiting. In the very, very rare case of a significant head injury, the baby may seem okay until the swelling inside her head exceeds the capacity of the pop-off and she develops severe life-threatening symptoms. This is really rare but is the reason that your pediatri-

## ITTY-BITTY BABIES

Newborns and very young infants are more difficult to examine after a head injury and are more likely to have CT scanning or further testing after a fall or head injury. There are a few reasons for this, starting with the fact that newborns have skulls that are not as thick and strong as an older baby's and are more easily injured. Tiny babies also aren't very easy to evaluate. Is he lying there like a lump because he's a week old or because he injured his head?

cian may be more likely to want to see a young baby after a bonk to the head.

For older babies and little kids with a head injury, if the child is awake and alert, and is back to his normal self (after the obvious period of crying and comforting, followed by distraction with a new toy and a cookie), things are most likely fine. If over the next few hours he remains his usual self and is eating and drinking normally, things are good. You are welcome to give your pediatrician a call (during normal business hours), but it is likely that all you will receive is reassurance.

After a kid has sustained a blow to the head, acting a little cranky can be normal. He might have a headache, so an appropriate dose of pain medicine would be good. A child who has recently suffered a head injury might be a little sleepier or more listless than usual, but don't worry as long as you can wake him easily and he is behaving relatively normally.

## WHEN TO CALL THE DOCTOR

Repeated, discrete episodes of vomiting (more than three to four times), acting weird or inappropriate, and extreme sluggishness or sleepiness following a head injury are all reasons to give your doctor a quick call. A bruise or "bump" generally isn't, unless she's a very young infant (under three months).

*Swelling.* There are a lot of blood vessels in the face and scalp, so it is not at all uncommon for a baby or child to have pretty impressive swelling and bruising after a head injury. A large bruise or swelling is *not* generally a reason to send a child to the ER or to order an X-ray study. As I've said over and over, it is more important to watch your child's behavior and temperament than to fixate on the size of the lump on her head. Remember, her head is hard. The skin is loose. The blood vessels are many. So an impressive swelling of the face, around the eye, or on the scalp is pretty common. That said, the younger the infant (less than six months), the more careful we are. Any child who has hit the *back* of his head and then develops black eyes or bruising behind the ears should be evaluated. If you are at all in doubt, call your pediatrician, but remember that really scary bumps on the head after a fall are very rarely anything about which you should worry.

## THE GUSHY SPOT

After a bump to the head, a fair amount of swelling, or a "knot," is quite normal. After several days, the knot might begin to feel very soft or even liquid as the blood slowly turns from a clot back into fluid and leaves the area. Don't worry about it.

*Vomiting.* Everyone is worried about vomiting after a head injury. It is important here to distinguish between the vomiting that occurs right after the fall, while the child is hysterical and crying, gagging on his tears, and eventually making himself throw up, and the vomiting that occurs minutes to hours *after* a head injury. Vomiting one or two times in the immediate period after hitting her head is not unusual. However, vomiting can be a sign of increased pressure around the brain, so we would start to worry if the vomiting continues or occurs much later, after everyone has calmed down. I usually tell parents that more than three to four episodes of vomiting, or vomiting that is occurring well after the excitement of the fall, is of concern and the child should definitely be examined urgently. While the vomiting may be a sign of a simple concussion (or entirely coincidental with the start of a stomach bug), we want to be very sure that there is no increased pressure from a bruise or bleeding inside the skull.

*Sleeping.* He can go to sleep after hitting his head. The need to keep an injured child awake is a fantastic myth that has been perpetuated by some really bad television. It's not the falling asleep that is important; it is whether a child can be woken easily, and whether his sleepiness is normal for that time of day. Too many parents proudly deny their child his afternoon nap after a head injury, making him an irritable, sleepy wreck. No one can know if he's acting that way because he missed his nap or because of the injury! If he wants to sleep, let him. If it makes you feel better to wake him up every few hours during the night, go ahead. He doesn't have to have a conversation with you, just make sure he can be easily aroused and then let him go back to sleep. If he is sleeping for a very long time at a time of day when he normally would be awake, check that he can be aroused and then give your doctor a call to talk it over.

*Is an X-Ray Necessary?* If your pediatrician sends your family to the emergency room, your child will be examined and the decision to get a cat scan, or computerized tomography (CT) scan, will be made based on several factors, including the child's age, the type of injury, her physical exam, and any symptoms she may be having. Insisting on a CT scan when the physician recommends against it is not a good idea, for many reasons including nonessential radiation exposure. More information on the risks of radiation and the reasons for and against a CT scan in kids is found in Chapter 15. However, if your kid does need a scan, she should absolutely get one. As for X-rays of the skull, these are indicated only in very small infants under certain circumstances or in specialized cases, such as when looking for gun shrapnel. In older babies and young children, routine skull X-rays after a head injury are generally not indicated (although there have been a couple of times when even I have ordered them). Therefore, there may be instances when a physician will want a skull X-ray, so don't argue with her, but understand that this is not commonly done. The information they give us is not nearly as important as our physical exam. If we are worried about injury to the brain, a CT scan is the test of choice, as the X-rays will tell us nothing about bleeding and brain injury.

Even with a normal CT scan, children may continue to have some symptoms, such as difficulty concentrating or headaches, for a couple of weeks thereafter. Whether an X-ray or a CT scan is performed or not, you should absolutely learn about the late signs of a head injury, watch your child, and return to the hospital if needed.

## How Long Am I Benched?

When a kid has suffered a head injury, a good rule of thumb is to try to avoid another one in the near future. This means no sports until a minimum of one week without any symptoms has passed. Your pediatrician should clear him for a return to full activity. For a little kid, this might mean some quieter play indoors for a few days. It is extremely rare, but a second strong blow to the head before the brain has had time to recover from the last insult can be devastating.

### Headache

It can be very difficult to know if your baby or small child has a headache. Infants may swat at their heads because they have an earache or a headache, or because they are bored. In general, "headache" is a pretty unusual complaint in a baby.

As a toddler, however, he may be able to verbalize the fact that his head hurts. Whether you are worried because she's using her head for batting practice, or your toddler has been whining all day, you want to know when to worry or not.

Babies and young children have a great deal of difficulty localizing pain. They may complain of wrist pain when they have an elbow injury, for instance. Older children are often better at describing the location of pain, but still may have trouble describing the type and intensity of what ails them. There are many, many reasons why a child may appear to have a headache. Several infections, such as viruses or strep throat, classically cause a headache, even though the infection is *not* in any way spreading into the brain.

Fever is another common cause of headaches. For most children, if you suspect a headache, a size-appropriate dose of pain reliever, such as ibuprofen or acetaminophen, is reasonable and should relieve their symptoms.

So when do we want to know about a headache? First, a child with a fever and a severe headache that does not improve when the fever goes down, especially if it is accompanied by listlessness or irritability, crying when the child is picked up or moved, or a stiffness of the neck or body, should be seen urgently. In a child without a fever, we are more concerned about the frequency and duration, as well as the timing, of headaches. A physician should see a child who is having daily headaches, especially upon awakening, or headaches accompanied by vomiting. A headache that wakes a child from sleep, or one that worsens with changes in position (like from sitting to lying down), is also concerning. In addition, a baby or child who seems to have weakness of an arm or leg, or who is unable to do things she could do before, such as pull to a stand or walk, should be seen in an urgent fashion.

WRITE IT DOWN

If your child is having frequent headaches, keeping a headache diary (recording day of week, time of day, activity, duration, and what made it better) can be immensely helpful to your pediatrician. You should also jot down any symptoms associated with the headache, such as sensitivity to light, nausea or vomiting, and the like.

## The Soft Spot Is Too Soft/Full/Big/Little

Remember, from Chapter 1, why we have soft spots when we are born? Recall that in order for us to squeeze our big brains down the birth canal, we have to be born while we are still relatively small and immature. Thus, the helpless baby. What's more, our brains are going to continue to grow after we are born, so the bones of our skull must be able to move and grow accordingly. Hence the soft spot. In medical terms, the soft spot is called the anterior fontanel. It is the meeting point of two bones of the skull, which will, over time, grow together until they fuse into a solid skull.

As for whether the soft spot seems flat, sunken, or full, if little Franklin is smiling and cooing, it's probably fine. A very

HOW BIG FOR HOW LONG?

The time frame for these bones to close over the soft spot has a very wide range, but most are closed by fifteen to eighteen months. So, if you think the soft spot is still there after the age of two, don't just cover it with a hair ribbon, tell somebody. As for how big or small a fontanel should be, they will get a bit bigger before closing up and it's most likely normal. Your pediatrician can tell you.

sunken fontanel may signal dehydration in some infants, but that baby won't be smiling at you. The same goes for a very full or bulging soft spot. This could signal increased pressure around the brain and needs to be evaluated. On the other hand, if it just bulges up when she is screaming mad and then goes right back to normal, don't give it another thought. A soft spot that appears to be bulging all the time needs to be evaluated (during regular business hours). As always, if she is acting her normal self, happy and smiley, there is no emergency.

And yes, you can wash a soft spot. You can comb over a soft spot. You can put your fingers on it. You won't poke his brain out. You aren't even touching his brain. You are touching skin and fat and thick membranes and fluid and everything else that protects his little brain from curious people like you.

## Is His Head Supposed to Look Like That?

So you got over the shock of the misshapen newborn head, and after a week or so under that hat, everything smoothed out and started looking pretty normal. But now you are starting to worry again. One side looks funny. The back looks too flat. His head is looking mighty big. So what is normal?

Remember that we have several plates in our skull that aren't fully stuck to one another until many months after birth. If a baby spends all his time on his back, or with his head turned a certain way, it is possible for the plates on one side to grow a bit flatter than on the other side. You should try your best to make sure that wee Justin doesn't spend too much time in any one position. Don't become obsessed with moving his head every ten minutes. Just don't leave him on his back twenty-four hours a day.

TUMMY TIME

Remember, a baby should always sleep on her back. But when awake, make sure she gets some supervised time lying on her tummy. Not only is it good for her development if she gets to look around and use different muscles, but she'll give her hair and skull a chance to even themselves out. A flat, bald posterior is silly looking.

Rarely, some of the plates in the skull may begin to stick, or fuse, together too early. This condition is called craniosynostosis and is very, very rare. When this happens, the other plates must spread out farther, to accommodate that growing brain. The result is that a baby's head may look misshapen or uneven. If you are worried about this, call your pediatrician, who can determine if this is true closure of the bones or not. It may be necessary to have some X-ray studies done and possibly get a referral to a specialist. Same for babies who seem to have an awfully big head. Your doctor should be measuring your baby's head, along with her height and weight, at her checkups. By following the growth of the head on a special chart, we can reassure ourselves that the baby's head is growing at the same rate as the rest of him. However, in a rare condition, called hydrocephaly, too much of the fluid that bathes our brain begins to build up, which can cause pressure on the brain. Because babies have skulls that can still grow, this might cause a faster rate of growth of the skull than we would like. If you think your baby's head seems to be too large, or is growing more quickly than the rest of him, please ask your doctor to take a look. Chances are that he just inherited a big noggin from the "other" side of the family. Seriously, we call this familial macrocephaly, and it just means that everyone in the family wears a bigger-than-average hat size. An inherited big head is definitely more common than hydrocephaly, but you want to be sure.

## The Nervous System

### The Jittery Baby

Allow me to reassure you that all babies and little kids have funny little twitches and odd movements that they make, often while sleeping. If you are worried that the movements seem very large or happen too frequently, set up a video camera. No matter how well you describe the movements, capturing a few on video will make your pediatrician's assessment a million times easier. In a few seconds, she can reassure you that the movements are normal and he's not actually having a seizure.

Seizures, when they do happen, are due to abnormal electrical activity in the brain. The lightning storm causes symptoms dependent upon the location of the abnormal electrical impulses. If the entire brain is involved, the whole body will be involved. If only a small portion of the brain is involved, only the part of the body for which that area of the brain is responsible will have abnormal activity.

If your baby or child does seem to be having a seizure, look to see if he is awake and alert. A generalized seizure, which is a rhythmic jerking of the whole body, is the most common type of seizure in children after the newborn period and may have many causes. A child who is having a generalized seizure will *not* be alert and looking around. Other types of seizures may involve just one part or side of the body and the kid may or may not be awake. In general, we tend to worry a bit more about the seizures that don't involve the entire body. If you think your child is having a seizure, and she does not stop on her own within a few minutes, is turning blue, or is unconscious, go ahead and call for an ambulance. Young infants with seizures should also be seen more urgently. If she has a seizure and stops on her own, returning to normal within a few minutes, it is okay to call your pediatrician before dialing 911. As with jittery young infants, if your baby or young child is having frequent episodes of odd behavior that you think could be an unusual type of seizure, grab your video camera. Get it on film and take the footage to your pediatrician's office. A real-life movie of the moment in question is worth a thousand trips to the ER after the fact.

For a discussion of febrile seizures, or seizures with a fever, see Chapter 10.

## How to Help During a Seizure

If a child (or anyone else for that matter) is having a seizure, you do *not* need to give mouth-to-mouth. CPR is for blue and floppy, not blue and seizing. Also, please do *not* put anything in her mouth. She will not choke on her tongue, but she sure might have trouble breathing around your wallet! Most parents panic during a seizure and call for help immediately, but it is okay to wait a few moments for the seizure to stop (if you can keep your cool), then call your pediatrician afterward. Call 911 if the seizure does not stop within a few (five) minutes. Once the seizure stops, you can turn the child onto his side to help him breathe more easily until he is fully awake.

## Weakness

It is most important to differentiate between the kind of "weakness" my husband develops when it is time to do the dishes and true weakness, meaning a loss of muscle strength or paralysis of the nerves. Many parents complain that their child is "weak," but this is often in the setting of a viral illness, dehydration, or fever, and when given a little fluid and acetaminophen or ibuprofen, little Tatum goes right back to her usual, destructive self. However, true muscle weakness or lack of movement is very concerning to us.

### Going Backward

Any baby or small child who seems to be *losing* skills that she had a week ago needs to be seen by her doctor urgently.

An infant who seems to have generalized weakness, has difficulty feeding, and is much floppier than she was a few days ago needs to be seen urgently. In rare circumstances, infants can be infected with botulism. Older children and adults are able to ingest the botulism bacteria without trouble because our immune systems are more developed. However, smaller babies can become infected. The spores that cause this infection can be found in honey and corn syrup, which is why babies under age one should stick to regular sugar. Botulism causes weakness of all the muscles of the body, including those that help us breathe. Fortunately the infection can be treated, and the earlier it is diagnosed, the better. Treatment stops progression of the disease but doesn't reverse the weakness; babies will slowly regain use of their muscles and have an excellent chance for a full recovery. However, while they are ill, we may need to support their breathing and help them to get enough fluid and calories.

A baby or child who has weakness of one side of the body, or one arm or leg, is also worrisome and needs to be seen immediately. A sudden limp, or falling to one side when she could sit perfectly unsupported a week ago, is certainly of concern. If your child seems to be losing her "milestones" in development, or you are concerned about any abnormality of her strength, call your pediatrician.

## Behavior

### Colic

Colic is just so frustrating, I want to scream. Colic is a condition where a baby, usually starting around two weeks of age and continuing until about three months, cries for several hours a day, without any explanation. Evening and late-night or early morning crying is common, although he might wail the whole day through.

Some babies with colic are soothed by loud noises or by rhythmic movements, such as (while properly restrained in an infant car seat) riding in a car or sitting on top of a washing

### IT'S NOT GAS

Grandma will tell you that gas and stomach pains cause colic. People think this is because babies with colic tend to tense up their bellies and pull up their legs when they cry, and they might toot a lot. But research has shown that colic is more about having an immature nervous system, which leads to a fussy, out-of-control baby. The screaming infant then swallows a lot of air, giving her gas, and she tenses up her belly because it allows her to belt it out with more ferocity. Colic disappears right around the same time that a baby learns to smile and hold her head up and begins to interact with the world like a somewhat intelligent being, thus confirming that an immature brain is the source of the trouble.

machine. There are several other things that parents can do to soothe their infant and I will shamelessly plug a book by a man named Dr. Harvey Karp called *The Happiest Baby on the Block*. Dr. Karp isn't giving me anything—in fact, he doesn't even know me and probably doesn't want to be associated with me, but I'm just telling you what I tell every other family that comes into the ER. This is the book I buy for all of my friends who are expecting. Dr. Karp's book gives several strategies for calming a crying infant and I won't go over them all here. But let me tell you what happened last time I saw a "crying infant." Picture a full ER on a very busy evening. All my rooms were full and the family of a three-week-old who was screaming bloody murder was huddled in the corner, looking frazzled, embarrassed, and exhausted. Now, I felt for them, but really, I felt more for myself. Screaming babies are annoying. So I grabbed a blanket, and while quickly introducing myself and apologizing to the family (and the other ten patients waiting with them) for the long wait, swaddled that baby tightly, flipped her over, and began rhythmically patting her on the back while swinging her to and fro. Instant silence. Mom burst into tears and the waiting room applauded. It has never failed me. Go buy his book.

## But He's Not Normally Such a Crybaby

When an infant isn't normally "colicky" but is just screaming for no apparent reason and acting entirely out of character, I run through my quick crying checklist. First, an infant with extreme irritability in the setting of fever or other symptoms, such as vomiting, should be evaluated. Second, check the fingers and toes and, if there is one, the penis, because occasionally a strand of hair can become caught around one of these appendages and create a tourniquet-like effect, essentially strangulating the affected part. This needs to be dealt with immediately by either cutting the hair or using a hair-removing product such as Nair, but unless you are five hundred miles from the nearest medical attention and it's snowing, this is best left to a medical professional. Third, there may be a scratch on the eyeball called a corneal abrasion. This can happen when an active baby swipes his eye inadvertently (because he's not old enough to have intent or self-injurious behavior) and scratches his cornea. This hurts a whole lot, but heals up often within twenty-four hours. To find the scratch, a little dye is placed into the eye and then the baby is held under a blacklight to look for any irregularities of the cornea. Clearly, you cannot be doing this at home. Even if you own a disco parlor. This diagnosis is made in the ER or at your doctor's office. A soothing ointment to protect the eye until the scratch has healed will often be prescribed. Finally, one crying infant came to our emergency room because he had been screaming the entire day. The nurse took off his shoes and he suddenly let out a sigh and quieted down. They were new shoes. And they were too tight. So, quickly, before heading to the emergency room, strip down your youngster and make sure there are no diaper pins poking him, that his skin isn't stuck in a zipper, and that his shoes aren't pinching his little piggies.

## Toddler Weirdness

Older babies and toddlers will do some really weird things. Some of them are subconscious, others are attention-seeking behaviors, and some start out as unintentional behaviors but carry on because of the attention generated. If your child is doing something really odd but can be distracted or seems to find it fun, especially when she sees your face, you need to ignore it. I know a toddler whose current fun game is to suddenly act petrified. Her family is convinced she is either seeing ghosts or having seizures and begin yelling and carrying on when she does this. So then she laughs. And the cycle continues. If you are really concerned, call your doctor.

## Head Banging

It is not uncommon for an older baby or young toddler to develop a nasty habit of banging his head against the nearest solid object. Naturally, his parents freak out and try to do anything they can think of to keep him from hitting his poor little head. Because little Bobby is obviously going to give himself brain damage, right? Wrong. Some little kids find the repeated movement of banging their heads to be a sort of self-soothing exercise, like a yoga mantra. Some little ones will do it more when they are tired or irritable, or during a tantrum. Because they are hitting their own heads, they won't hit hard enough to cause any damage, no matter what you think. The moment it hurts, he will back off. I have never seen, nor heard of, a child giving himself a serious head injury by banging.

What is important for you to know is that this is a normal little kid behavior. He probably doesn't even realize what he is doing. Until you freak out and make a big deal of it. And then it becomes a game, or even worse, a power struggle. The bigger deal you make of it, the more attention he gets, the more he bangs his head. Ignore him.

If, however, your child is not normally a head-banger, new banging may be a response to pain, such as from an earache. And if he is still banging away after the age of three, or you are concerned that there are other issues with his development or sociability, give your pediatrician a call.

## Night Terrors

Toddlers and young children may experience a phenomenon known as "night terrors." Imagine you are on your way to bed, having just finished that pint of mint chip, when your peacefully sleeping child begins to scream. And not just a little peep. We are talking the hellish, I'm being attacked, panicked kind of yelling. So you drop the spoon and race upstairs, only to find that she is actually kind of still asleep. Asleep and screaming. So you grab her and start yelling and then she wakes up and becomes truly terrified, because her frightened parents are standing over her, making noise and shaking her awake.

Night terrors are a type of abnormal sleep, like sleepwalking or talking in your sleep. Night terrors are different from bad dreams in that there isn't really a bad dream happening. Kids with night terrors have no memory of the event and can't recall a scary dream. The only person who is traumatized the next morning is the parent. As scary as these events are for you, please know that this phase is only temporary. You can probably settle her back down with a few gentle words and a rearrangement of her blankets. There is no reason to wake her completely up if she calms and resumes sleeping. Then you can go slip yourself a cocktail and prepare yourself for the next one. Most little kids will average one episode a week until they outgrow this annoying phase.

## Parental Behavior

Babies and little kids can be really frustrating. They don't listen, they are emotionally labile, they can't be reasoned with or even bribed. It's a tough job, policing a kid who doesn't know any better but seems to be on a permanent path to self-destruction. Older toddlers might have a better understanding of what goes and what doesn't and might respond to outright bribery, but they are still egocentric little beasts, determined to battle for control of any situation.

Kids respond well to consistency and repetition. Don't be afraid to set boundaries. Use positive reinforcement, such as praise or rewards, to help guide your kid's behavior. Try to be conscious of what is an age-appropriate expectation of your child. A six-month-old doesn't know that you don't squawk in church, any more than a three-year-old can be expected to sit through a four-course fine dining experience.

All that aside, if you feel your buttons have been pushed just one too many times, or if you don't think you can stand one more second of crying, ask for help and get yourself together. Go into another room. Take a breath. Call your mom, your pediatrician, or your best friend. I would rather see you in my ER at 2 a.m. because you just can't take it anymore than I would ever want to see another shaken baby or knocked-around toddler.

# seeing and hearing

## The Eyes and Ears

This chapter is about two of the most important sensory organs of the head and neck: the eyes we see with and the ears with which we hear. They are pretty important organs and problems are usually pretty apparent. Even if Little Red Riding Hood's grandma totally missed the fact that her granddaughter was a wolf, she did, after all, comment on her eyes. Let's talk about the normal, the not-so-normal, and what to do if one of these organs is injured. Like when her brother tries to poke her eye out.

### The Eyes

#### Crusty or Red Eyes

We all have little tubes that lead from the inner corner of our eyes into our nose. This is partly why our nose runs when we cry. Without these little tubes, the normal tears that keep our eyes nice and lubricated would be streaming down our face all day long. However, in some babies, this tube is not fully open at birth and you may find yourself with a baby who seems to constantly have crusty and draining eyes. Most often this tube will open up by itself by one year of age. If not, an eye doctor may need to help it along, but this is pretty rare. You can encourage the tube to open up by gently massaging along the area just inside the eye and onto the bridge of the nose. Your pediatrician can teach you how to do this properly. Otherwise, just wipe the drainage and crusts off with a warm washcloth as needed (e.g., just before taking pictures). As long as the drainage does not become very thick and green or yellow in color and the white part of the eye is not red, it is not an infection and just annoying. However, should you think that the eye is becoming more red or inflamed looking, or should the drainage change in quality, please call your doctor.

The dreaded pink eye is the other cause of a red, draining eye. Pink eye, or conjunctivitis, is an infection of the conjunctiva, or linings of the eyelids. Itching, pain, watering, and drainage that is white, green, yellow, or even sometimes bloody can occur. Both viruses (more commonly) and bacteria cause pink eye, and it is often difficult to tell the difference. For newborns, bacterial pink eye is considered an emergency, but for older babies and young children, there isn't great evidence that bacterial conjunctivitis needs to be treated in an otherwise healthy kid. Then again, many physicians will treat a presumed bacterial infection with antibiotic drops. For one thing, daycares won't accept a kid back until he is on drops. This is, of course, ridiculous; most cases are caused by a virus and won't become less contagious with medication, but hey, why fight the inane? What I tell parents when diagnosing their child with pink eye is that I'm giving them the eye drops in case it is a bacteria (when I don't know), and that it will either get better in three to four days with the drops or five to seven days by itself. The most important thing is to *wash your hands*, because conjunctivitis is extremely contagious and will spread through your family, school, and neighborhood like wildfire. Because children can't help touching their eyes when they are hurting and goopy, and then they go around touching everything else. As for actually helping your child, a warm wet washcloth will wash away the mucus and may help with the irritation and keep him from rubbing his eyes. Other than that, remember that pink eye looks horrible, but it will go away and is probably far more bothersome to you and his teacher than to the actual kid.

### Age Alert!

Pink eye, or conjunctivitis, in newborn babies (twenty-eight days and younger), as opposed to everyone else, is considered serious because some infections acquired at birth may cause eye infections that permanently affect a baby's vision. These infections can occur within a few days or a couple of weeks. Occasionally the duct itself will become infected and will appear red and swollen and may require antibiotic therapy. Should you think that the eye is becoming redder or more inflamed looking, or should the drainage change in quality, please call your doctor.

If the skin around the eye becomes swollen or red, particularly if your child is acting more ill, with fever or vomiting, or if the eye seems to be poking out a bit from the face, this should be seen rather urgently. An older child may complain that it hurts to move his eyeball and this should prompt a quick phone call to your doctor. While it may just be an infection of the skin around the eye, which will respond to antibiotics by mouth, sometimes the infection can spread into the space behind the eye and be a real problem. It can be difficult to tell the difference, so let your doctor know if the eye begins to look any worse.

## You'll Poke Your Eye Out!

I have never actually seen a child who has poked his eye out. But we do see plenty of kids with eye injuries of various sorts in the emergency room. If your child has suffered trauma to the eye, be it self-inflicted or someone else's fault, don't panic.

For blunt trauma to the skin around the eye, such as getting accidentally hit with a toy, if there is a cut, or laceration, in the skin around the eye or eyelids, this may need to be repaired. Any cuts that actually go through the edges of the eyelids will probably need to be repaired by an eye doctor. Most cuts will likely need emergency care and you should call your doctor. If there is just a scrape, or abrasion, of the skin, there is nothing to be done, and a little antibiotic ointment and a bandage will suffice. For bruising of the skin (a "black eye"), be sure that the eyeball itself moves in all directions and without pain. You can dance from side to side and wave a puppet while someone else holds your baby's head still to make sure the eyeball moves. If all seems okay, nothing other than cold packs (if she'll tolerate them) and pain medicine are needed. An injured eye can become very swollen and bruised

## SWELLING SHUT

Eyes are surrounded by a lot of loose skin that can hold a lot of blood and fluid and can become very swollen or very bruised much more easily than other parts of our body where the skin is pulled a bit tighter. So an eye can look like it sustained an insult *far* worse than the actual injury.

in a short period of time. The bruising will gradually change in color and fade, although this may take several weeks.

As for the actual eyeball, or globe, see if it appears normal. Look at the colored part (the iris) and the black circle (the pupil). These should appear to be perfectly circular (unless your child was born with an abnormality of either, in which case you should already know this). Any abnormality in the shape of either should prompt urgent evaluation.

Assuming that there are no obvious injuries to the eyelids or eye itself, it is now okay to observe your child for a while. If he seems to be very irritable, crying, rubbing at his eye, or in pain, it is possible that he may have a small scratch across the eye, called a corneal abrasion. An abrasion, or scrape, of the cornea is extremely painful. A kid with a corneal abrasion will keep that eye closed and be very unhappy. These scratches cannot be seen with the naked eye, but you might find (if she'll open it!) that the eye looks red and irritated. Fortunately, most heal up within twenty-four hours. Although there is no specific treatment for a corneal abrasion, save perhaps a soothing antibiotic ointment, we do want to see these kids promptly. This is because we (1) want to know that a small abrasion truly is responsible for his crying and (2) need to ensure that appropriate follow-up is arranged, to ensure the abrasion heals in a timely fashion without complication. In addition, a corneal abrasion may result from a foreign body stuck on the underside of the upper eyelid, scraping along the eyeball every time he blinks; we need to look under the eyelid if the scratch pattern looks suspicious. Perhaps more important, we can actually make your child feel a little bit better. Numbing eye drops take away all the pain and allow for a much easier examination of a child's eye. While we can't send you home with the drops, because a numb eye is an easily injured eye, we can grant little Frankie a reprieve from his misery. Furthermore, most doctors will prescribe antibiotic drops or ointment to prevent an infection in the scratch. A nice thick ointment is not only easier to use in babies and children, but can also be very soothing to a sore eyeball.

In essence, if your child has suffered an eye injury and you are worried in any way that she seems to be in pain or having difficulty seeing, call your pediatrician promptly. No one is going to dismiss concerns for an injury that may threaten a child's vision and we would rather be safe than sorry.

## There's Glitter in Her Eye!

When I was in training, we spent an entire morning practicing removing glitter from a cow eyeball. Because you never know when you are going to need *that* skill. Seriously, children do put things in their eyes, often unintentionally, and this situation may be difficult to handle at home. If you see glitter, for instance, or some other foreign-looking item on the eyeball, do *not* attempt to remove it with your finger. First, you can try pulling the upper eyelid gently over the lower eyelid, which will probably make her eyes water, washing away the offending material. If that doesn't work, gently flush water over her face and eyes for about five or ten minutes and take another look. If it is still there, you are probably going to have to see a professional.

Let's say little Jack has been playing with Daddy's hammer and flattening all of Mommy's copper jewelry. And then he begins to complain of eye pain. In any circumstance where we think a foreign body, in particular metal, may have flown into the eye after being hit or otherwise broken, we want to see those kids right away. Even if everything looks okay, a small piece of fast-flying metal can penetrate the eyeball and cause serious injury.

## RINSE FIRST, TALK LATER!

If she's poured glass cleaner or some other household product into her eye, get her to the sink as fast as you can and run her eyes under water for at least twenty minutes. You can also pour water from a cup or bottle, or use the saline solution in which you store your contacts. After a good rinse, you or someone else should look at the bottle to see if there are any instructions and call your local Poison Center or your pediatrician. Some things are quite harmless, albeit painful, like soap. Other chemicals may cause serious burns to the eye and will need rapid treatment. The most effective way to prevent injury to the eye after exposure to a chemical is a really good rinse with water. After you have done the initial rinse, the local Poison Center will be able to tell you whether your child will need further care at the emergency room. If sent to the hospital, your child will likely have her eyes rinsed thoroughly again, and afterward we can check the acidity of her tears to make sure that all traces of the chemical are gone. Unfortunately, even the best and most rapid intervention can't prevent all injury to the eye, so any evidence of injury or a burn will need to be followed up by an eye doctor.

## Bumpy Eyes

If you spot a lump on the upper or lower eyelid, don't panic. The most common eyelid bump is a stye, which is just a little infected pimple of the eyelid. Pimples and styes are formed when normal bacteria on the body get trapped inside the skin and want to get out. Swelling, pain, and pus are normal. Styes can be quite painful and may become large and red. As long as it is just the bump that is growing in size and redness, and not the whole eyelid, not to worry. Warm compresses (a hot, damp washcloth will work) encourage the stye to drain. Don't be alarmed if green or yellow pus comes out from the inside of the eyelid.

### EMERGENCY!

Any type of rash or bumps around the eye that look like little blisters should be seen more urgently, especially if the child or anyone in the family has cold sores. Your pediatrician may decide that a referral to an ophthalmologist, or eye doctor, is necessary. The herpes virus that causes cold sores can sometimes cause an infection in the eye that can permanently affect vision.

Another type of eyelid bump is called a chalazion, which can also be painful and red and tends to hang around a bit longer or recur. This bump is different from a stye because it sits farther back on the eyelid, rather than just on the edge of the lashes. The eye itself is not in danger in any way, but chalazions can be annoying and ugly. They sometimes need referral to an eye doctor if they become chronic (i.e., they don't go away within a couple of weeks or recur).

## Eye Pain

If your baby or child is acting as if her eye hurts, is rubbing at it or otherwise indicating that she is uncomfortable, you probably need to call your pediatrician. There are many reasons for pain in the eye, the most common being a small scratch along the surface of the eye, called a corneal abrasion. In fact, when evaluating an infant for unexplained crying, we examine the eyes specifically for such an injury.

## Subconjunctival Hemorrhage

A large red area on the white part of the eyeball is called a subconjunctival, or scleral, hemorrhage. This is simply a broken blood vessel overlying the sclera, or white part, of the eye. Anyone can get this after coughing vigorously, vomiting, or laughing hysterically. Anything that causes increased pressure in your face can make one of these little vessels burst. Coughing until you puke can do it. Getting poked in the eye by your big sister can do it. It will go away by itself. Don't look at it. Don't worry about it.

## Strabismus

Lots of babies are cross-eyed. By six months, this should straighten out. If not, then your pediatrician should send you to an ophthalmologist. Scheduling an appointment with an eye doctor sooner than six months is likely a waste of your time. Also, some babies have a fold of skin on either side of their nose that makes them look cross-eyed when they aren't. Your pediatrician should be able to tell the difference between a baby that truly has strabismus (crossed eyes or a "lazy" eye) and pseudostrabismus (he's faking it). Just kidding, he's not faking it on purpose. But it's not a true crossed eye. Your doctor can easily distinguish between the two.

## The Red Reflex

If you ever think your kid is going to outgrow the need to have all his pictures Photoshopped, think again. That devilish red light in his eyes is here to stay. We call this redness the red reflex and it is a sign of a healthy retina. Any change in the appearance of the baby's eye demands an urgent appointment with your pediatrician. So if you notice while playing that one eye seems cloudy or white, or if in a picture only one eye is red, call your doctor. If it only happens in one out of a hundred photos, it is probably nothing, but you need your doctor to take a look.

## The Ears

### Pulling on the Ears

A baby usually pulls on her ears because they are attached to the sides of her head and she is bored and found a cool new plaything. Pulling on the ears does not always mean there is an infection. However, swatting at or pulling on an ear, when combined with cold symptoms, fever, vomiting, or fussiness, may indicate an infection of the inner ear. Or it may not. Otalgia means ear pain without an infection. Just having a cold may cause pressure and pain when no infection exists. The official name for an infection of the inner part of the ear is otitis media. And, oh boy, is otitis media a hot topic among pediatricians. First, it can be pretty hard to tell if an ear is infected or not, even when looking directly at the eardrum with one of our doctor toys. Second, many people will argue that most cases of otitis media do not require treatment with antibiotics. In fact, in many countries, doctors will wait several days after making the diagnosis before starting treatment to see if a child will improve by himself. There are many reasons why this approach has solid merit, but I won't go into a detailed discussion here. Rather, you should take from this the point that an ear infection is not necessarily a condition that requires emergency treatment with antibiotics. Whether your child's pain is due to otitis media or simple otalgia is irrelevant in the middle of the night. In either case, pain control is a must. Either acetaminophen or ibuprofen is fine. Eardrops that numb the eardrum are also available with a prescription from your doctor and might be something handy to have at home if your kid is prone to ear infections, saving you from a totally sleepless night until you can get to the pediatrician's office in the morning. As long as you can control your child's ear pain, there is no reason to run to the ER. Antibiotics won't make a difference on a short-term (one-day) basis, so other than controlling your child's pain, there is little that we in the emergency room can actually do.

## PULLING ON THE EARS

Kids pull on their ears for lots of reasons, only one of them being an infection. Even if there is an ear infection, the only treatment you need emergently is pain control. An appropriate dose of acetaminophen or ibuprofen should hold you until morning, when your doctor's office is open. Starting antibiotics in the middle of the night isn't going to make your kid stop crying!

Sometimes an eardrum that is infected will rupture, and pus and blood will come running out. This looks terrible, but actually can make your child feel much better since it is the pressure behind the infected eardrum that causes so much pain. Years ago doctors used to actually poke a hole in the drum on purpose to help relieve the misery. A ruptured otitis media may need antibiotic drops, but these can wait until morning. You should know that you did not cause the eardrum to rupture by waiting to have your child seen by a doctor. It is also very important that you do not put anything into the ear unless instructed by your pediatrician.

## WHAT NOT TO DO

If you are lucky enough to have the numbing eardrops for regular ear infections on hand, fantastic. But if there is pus or blood coming from the ear, assume that the eardrum has ruptured and don't use any numbing or pain drops. The medication may cause damage to the inside of the ear if put through an eardrum with a hole in it. Besides, the hole relieves the pressure and the pain should be all gone.

Most ruptured eardrums will heal up over time, although your doctor will want to check and make sure that it has done so. Very rarely a kid will need to see a specialist for repair.

What about airplane travel when your kid has an ear infection? Most of us will tell you that there are no absolutes, but remember that air travel can make a healthy set of ears hurt and pop. This will be worse if an ear is infected, and the change in air pressure may cause an intact eardrum to rupture, which would, of course, make your child feel instantly better. There is no right or wrong answer to this one. If you decide to fly, just arm yourself with a small (less than 90 ml) bottle of pain medicine in an FAA-approved plastic baggie.

## Earwax and Other Drainage

Our bodies produce earwax to protect the inside of our ears from people like you. Earwax, or cerumen, lines the ear canal, preventing dust and bugs and other stuff from settling there. The cerumen eventually works its way out of the ear and away from the body. Some kids produce a lot of earwax; others seem to make very hard wax that clogs up the ear canal. Earwax needs to be removed only if it is causing a problem. In the doctor's office, we use a little scoop to clear a path to see through, but you should never do this at home. It is too easy to poke a hole in the eardrum. If you are worried, you can purchase some over-the-counter earwax removal drops and use these. The drops, or even olive oil if you happen to be in the kitchen, will gradually soften the wax and let it drain out of the ear (and all over your bed linens). If you see some wax at the outer part of the ear, it is okay to take it off with your finger or a cotton swab, but never, ever put anything *into* the ear. You will only shove the wax in farther and might injure the delicate skin of the ear canal or the eardrum.

### IRRIGATE KINDLY

If you need to irrigate (wash out) your kid's ears for any reason, be forewarned that only room temperature water should be used. In medical school we learned about a cool brainstem reflex. Putting either warm or cold water in the ear forces the eyeballs to briefly look off to the side. Sounds fun but it will make you throw up.

## Do You Think, Maybe, I Should Put This Object in *Here*?

Kids are curious. They want to touch and explore everything. And they want to know, what will happen if they put a bean in their ear? Think of a possible hole on your kid's body where she potentially could try to stick something. I've got a story for it. So what do you do? Well, first, if you think that there is something somewhere that doesn't belong there, you're way ahead of the game. Most beads and Legos are removed from children's orifices during regular checkups. Whether you just suspect or can actually see something in one of your kid's ears, don't panic.

The only objects that need to come out on an emergent basis are things that could do damage if left in for too long. These include "vegetative" material (i.e., plants or food), such as popcorn or a dried bean. These objects may swell as they absorb fluid from the body and then become very difficult to remove. Another object that needs prompt removal is a disc battery. Batteries are dangerous because they may begin to leak some of the battery fluid, which can cause some serious damage to the body. If you aren't sure what your kid may or may not have stuck up his nose or in his ear, err on the side of caution and let your doctor know.

# bite and sniff

## The Nose, Mouth, and Throat

Now we come to the rest of the sensory organs of the head and neck: the nose we smell with, and the mouth and throat with which we taste the world around us. These are the components of the face that all empty into the same place and are connected in a way that allows us to blow milk out of our noses. What is normal, what isn't, and what do you do if he sticks a Lego up his nose?

### The Nose

### What's Up There?

Whether he got your cute little button nose or is stuck with Grandpa John's hook, there are just a couple of things you should know about his nose. First, those skin-colored fleshy lumps up inside there? They are called turbinates. They belong there. As for all the other things that are worrying you, let's attack them one by one.

### The Runny Nose

All babies sound congested. Most seem to become more congested as they get a little older. A newborn may sleep

## COLD MEDICINE

As discussed in Chapter 2, cough and cold medicines really aren't effective and most of us recommend *against* giving them to children. In fact, infant products are no longer available because of their lack of effectiveness and significant risk of side effects. They don't work and they can make your kid act way too sleepy or completely insane. What is just as effective, yet far safer, is a good home remedy. Stick ten beans in your pocket and throw one away every day. When the beans are gone, she'll be better.

soundly, but every five- to seven-week-old seems to have a "cold." There are many causes of a congested nose. In small babies, it is often just a buildup of mucus that can't easily be cleared. One tiny little boogie in a tiny little nose can make for a very noisy child, as the air tries to flow around through a very tiny tube with a very big obstruction. As they get bigger, so do their noses and everything quiets down. No worries. This bothers only you. As long as he is sleeping and eating without difficulty, not turning blue or seeming to open his mouth and gasp for air every few seconds, he's fine.

Regular baby congestion is not accompanied by a fever or difficulty breathing other than mild nasal congestion. Colds can cause fever. A cold, or upper respiratory infection, is a viral infection that attacks the nose and throat (upper airways) and causes mucus production and swelling. Allergies or environmental irritants don't cause a fever but may cause inflammation of the linings of the nose, leading to congestion and misery. So how do you know what is what?

A true viral upper respiratory infection generally begins with mild nasal congestion, progressing to thick yellow to

## THE BULB SYRINGE

Chances are you went home with a bulb syringe in your
hospital-provided postpartum gift pack. This is a wonderful
tool for getting mucus out of a baby's nose. Squeeze the
"bulb" end, put the tip gently into the baby's nose, and let the
bulb reexpand, hopefully sucking up some goobers and snot
along the way. However, please refrain from overzealous bulb
syringing. The constant pressure and irritation to the nose can
cause more irritation and swelling, making the situation even
worse. Control yourself. I should also point out that even
when done properly, using a bulb syringe may cause some
bleeding. As long as the bleeding stops in a little while, don't
worry. Just try to be really gentle.

green drainage and a loose cough. A fever may also be present
for the first few days. The snot eventually turns thick and
green and nasty before going away (or being replaced by a new
cold), in about ten days.

In older babies and young children, it can seem like every
week brings a new cold. Some kids, particularly those who are
in daycare or school (and therefore exposed to a lot of germs),
are constantly sick. Many parents are worried that their child

## SALINE DROPS

Try putting a few drops of saline (saltwater) solution in the
nose a couple of minutes before suctioning with a bulb
syringe to help loosen up the mucus. Store-bought saline is
fine, or you can mix 1/8 teaspoon salt in 8 ounces of water at
home. Make sure you don't reuse the solution and mix it up
fresh each time.

## THE COLOR OF SNOT

The color of the mucus your little one is blowing out his nose tells us *nothing* about whether the infection is caused by a bacteria or (most likely!) a virus. Antibiotics don't kill viruses, so they should not be prescribed just because of the color of the snot. Green, yellow, white, and bloody can all be the appearance of normal mucus developed during a cold.

has a weak immune system, but true immune problems are very, very rare, and they usually don't present themselves as one cold on top of another. Most children with immune system problems develop severe, life-threatening, or extremely unusual infections. A child with one upper respiratory infection after another is more likely simply picking up one germ after another. The *average* annual number of colds is around ten a year in *healthy* children! If it makes you feel better, there is evidence to suggest that these kids will probably have fewer illnesses as they grow older.

Maybe your kid just has allergies. While unusual in young infants, allergies may cause congestion or a chronically runny nose in toddlers and young children. While many kids with allergies have a parent or sibling with a history of the same, this is not at all required. One difference between allergies and colds is that the snot is generally more watery and white or clear in allergic kids. The big key is itchiness. Allergies cause itchiness, while a cold generally doesn't. So, if little Harry always seems to be rubbing his nose or eyes, or has a stuffy nose and red, watery eyes, you should definitely be thinking allergies. While cold medicines don't work, if you think your child may be having allergy symptoms, an over-the-counter allergy medicine for children is not an unreasonable thing to try. Unlike cold and cough medications, allergy medicines work. They contain drugs that have been shown to be effective for blocking the production of histamine, the hormone that causes allergic symptoms such as swelling and itchiness. For symptoms that can't be controlled with these medicines, speak to your pediatrician.

## No Operating Heavy Machinery

Most over-the-counter allergy medicines are safe for use in little kids and even infants. To be safe, read the label and check with your pediatrician if your little one is younger than a year or there is no infant dosing indicated. Be aware that some allergy medicines can cause sleepiness. But also be aware that *overstimulation* can occur with these same medicines, especially in young children. You might be expecting your two-year-old to drift off to sleep and will be horrified to find him bouncing from wall to wall.

How do you know if your child actually has a sinus infection, and not just a cold? Unfortunately, this is something that we pediatricians continue to argue about among ourselves. The sinuses are air pockets in the skull. Without them, our skulls would be solid bone and too heavy to lift off the pillow. These air pockets drain into the passages of the upper airways and can occasionally get infected. In children, the sinuses are not fully formed until about ten years of age; if a baby or child does get a sinus infection, it will be of the very small sinuses farther back in the skull. The bigger ones in the front of the face and above the eyes don't have air in them for several years after birth. With every cold, there is a fair amount of inflammation and mucus occurring within the sinuses. But a cold that doesn't go away after ten to fourteen days and seems to be actually worsening, with recurrence of fever and worsening congestion and nasal drainage, may represent a sinus infection that requires treatment with antibiotics. Pay attention. This is *very* different from a new cold that is following an old one. With a new cold, a kid will seem to get better and then a few days later begin again with watery congestion progressing to yellow and green. With a sinus infection, the old cold worsens and there is no reprieve. That means snot *every single day*, for *more than* ten to fourteen days before we are going to entertain the thought that this might be a bacterial superinfection. (Superinfection means that bacteria have infected something on top of an already present infection, like a cold. It doesn't mean that the infection is super or terribly powerful.) The difference is subtle; let your pediatrician be the final judge.

## THE MARATHON RUN

All little kids seem to have a perpetually runny nose. But if only one side is running, especially if it is particularly nasty looking or smells bad, either he or his sibling may have stuck something up there. And when I say "smells bad," I mean really, really bad. Can't go out in public bad. Needs three baths a day bad. Go read the section entitled "How about Putting Something in *Here?*" on page 98.

## The Nosebleed

If his nose begins to bleed, don't panic! It looks like more blood than it actually is. Even if it is all over his pillow and smeared across his face and into his hair. A little blood goes a long, long way. We all have little tiny blood vessels very close to the surface in the front part of our noses that can be easily damaged or irritated. The number one cause of nosebleeds in children is "digital trauma." Picking. And yes, he does. Everyone does. Even me. Other causes include nasal congestion for whatever reason, which can make the skin inside the nose more delicate and prone to bleeding. Very dry or cold air might dehydrate the skin inside the nose and lead to bleeding. Basically, anything that irritates the skin covering these vessels might make your nose bleed.

While more unusual in small infants, a nosebleed can happen to a child of any age. If your child's nose begins to bleed, sit him on your lap and gently squeeze the nostrils together with your fingers. If he'll allow it, he can lean slightly forward so that all that blood doesn't roll down his throat and into his tummy. Tipping his head back won't make the bleeding stop any faster and will fill his stomach with blood, Mother Nature's vomit inducer. The bleeding should stop within five or ten minutes. If it has stopped bleeding by then or isn't actively bleeding when you find your kid covered in blood, no more needs to be done. Just let your pediatrician know by phone if your infant (under one year) developed a bloody nose. Older kids, we're not generally so interested unless it is going on for a very long time (over a half hour) or is continually restarting to bleed. There are very, very rare conditions such as an abnormal artery or a problem with clotting of the blood that may present as a nosebleed. But again, these are really rare.

Some little kids get very frequent nosebleeds. If you are so lucky to get one of these children, speak to your pediatrician at your child's next checkup. Very rarely will there be a more serious explanation, such as high blood pressure or a bleeding abnormality. Some doctors will try to burn the little vessels in the nose to keep them from bleeding, using a substance called silver nitrate. While it looks pretty innocent, it can smart pretty badly and should be reserved only for those kids who truly have frequent, significant nosebleeds. Most kids simply need a little skin protection inside their delicate noses. A bit of petroleum jelly applied with a finger or cotton swab and nasal saline drops or spray are both good ways of keeping the nostrils moisturized and preventing nosebleeds. You can also try increasing the humidity in his room at night with a humidifier, but be certain to clean the device regularly, so that mold doesn't start growing inside the tank and make his allergies go haywire.

If your child develops a nosebleed that lasts longer than thirty minutes, is full of very large clots of blood, or he seems to be having trouble breathing, he should be seen immediately.

## PUKING BLOOD

When your nose bleeds, the blood runs down your throat and into your stomach and maybe even your lungs. So your kid might cough up a little blood after a nosebleed and this is okay. Blood does not sit well in anyone's tummy, so don't be surprised by a couple of episodes of bloody vomit.

## Trauma to the Nose

A blow to the nose can be pretty traumatic for everyone. To the victim, it can hurt like the dickens, and for everyone else the amount of blood can be quite scary. Relax. An injury to the nose is almost never an emergency.

For bleeding after a nose injury, gently pressing the nostrils together (as just recommended in "The Nosebleed," on page 95) should make the bleeding stop within ten minutes. If there is a cut of the skin across the nose, this may require sutures and you should check with your doctor. For all other injuries, expect a lot of pain and swelling. But rest assured, there is little reason to run out into the night seeking emergency care.

Parents seem to be most concerned about whether their child's nose is broken or not. The answer is, we probably can't say for sure. Injuries to the bones of the nose often involve the soft bone, or cartilage, which doesn't appear on an X-ray. Regardless, even if the nose is technically "broken," there is nothing to be done emergently. Only after the bruising and swelling have gone away will a plastic surgeon or ear, nose, and throat doctor attempt to realign a broken nose. While a nose is still swollen, it is impossible to know if the broken bone or cartilage has been set back into a normal position. Therefore, X-rays are of little to no use in the emergent evaluation of an injured nose. However, if the nose looks bent or crooked after the swelling has gone down, in about three to five days, you should ask your pediatrician about a referral to a specialist.

A bruise that develops along the inner part of the nose can compromise blood flow to the tissues of the nose, damaging the cartilage. This blood clot, a septal hematoma, looks like a blueberry inside the nose. Your doctor may want to take a peek up your kid's nose to make sure there is no hematoma, but these are very rare. If you happen to see a blue ball up there, call your doctor. In addition, if the nose continues to bleed heavily after applying pressure for ten to fifteen minutes, or your child has signs of other injuries, such as to the head, call your doctor urgently.

## How about Putting Something in *Here*?

Kids everywhere want to know. Does a Lego actually fit in a nostril? Do Barbie shoes? (The answer is yes.) Many parents don't even realize there is a bead in their kid's nose until it's seen by one of us. If there is something in your kid's nose that looks like it shouldn't be there, don't freak out. If she is a little baby, go find your three-year-old and ask him what he put in the baby's nose. If she is older and could have done this herself, don't get mad, she was only curious. Call your doctor.

## What Is That Smell?

If your kid develops a funny stench, give her the once-over. A piece of tissue up one nostril or some other foreign substance can cause a local collection of pus and goop, as the immune system tries to attack the foreign invader. Really stinky snot coming out one side of a child's nose should alert you to the possibility that your kid has stuck something up there that doesn't belong. The snot could be coming out of both sides, actually, depending on how much energy he invested.

As with foreign bodies in ears and other holes, the only objects that need to come out on an emergent basis are things that could become harmful if not removed. Plants or food, so-called vegetative materials, such as popcorn or a dried bean are on this list. Plant-based material may swell, making it very difficult to remove later. Magnets and disc batteries also should be removed promptly. Disc batteries can leak and cause serious local damage. Magnets are important when there is more than one, for example when two refrigerator magnets become stuck on either side of the middle section of the nose. When the magnets are being pulled toward one another, they can compress the skin and blood vessels and cause injury. Unfortunately, the magnets also seem to scoot rather far up into the nose, making removal an unpleasant and difficult task. I know.

## THE KISS

If you see something up your kid's nose, you can try a technique sometimes used in the ER called The Kiss. Pinch the empty side of the nose and cover his mouth with yours. Now blow. If you are lucky, the offending object will come flying out, spraying the side of your face with snot. Disgusting, but effective. Try this only once, and if you aren't successful, call your doctor.

## The Mouth, Inside and Out

### Sore Throat

Whether a sore throat is caused by an infection in the throat (bacterial or viral), blisters from a virus, or irritation from mucus and snot running down from above, most sore throats can be managed with pain control and fluids. Don't expect your baby to have the same enthusiasm for strained peas as she did last week. Encourage fluids and provide pain medication as needed.

Strep throat is a bacterial infection caused by the streptococcus bacteria. In older children, strep may cause fever, sore throat, swollen neck glands, headache, and even vomiting or belly pain. Younger kids may not have the classic symptoms of strep, but may have a sore throat, vomiting, or fever. It is very important to note that in kids older than preschool age, strep does *not* give you a runny nose. The diagnosis of strep throat should be made only when a throat swab is positive for the infection, because there are many, many causes of a fever and sore throat in kids (and adults!) and the vast majority are viral, meaning that antibiotics don't do a thing, except maybe cause an allergic reaction, create antibiotic resistance, or give your kid diarrhea and an ugly diaper rash. While the infection will go away by itself in about three to five days, strep throat is generally treated with antibiotics to prevent a very rare condition where the heart is damaged by the strep bacteria. This heart complication is called rheumatic fever, and should never be confused with the very common and harmless form of strep called scarlet fever. (For more on scarlet fever, see Chapter 9.) Rheumatic fever is incredibly rare nowadays but is the main reason we look for and treat strep throat.

## Is It Strep Throat?

Most sore throats are due to viral infections, like a simple cold. Antibiotics don't treat viruses. A runny nose and a cough make it *extremely* unlikely that a child has strep throat and needs antibiotics.

Children less than three don't generally need to be tested for strep. Babies and little kids can, rarely, get strep throat, usually from their older sibling or a pal at daycare. However, young children don't get the heart complications from strep throat, so there are very few times when a throat swab in a child under three years of age is indicated. There are situations where a doctor will want to test for and treat strep throat in a little one, so don't argue against it. Just realize that there is no real need for panic about strep in the very young.

In older kids, strep throat is treated with a course of antibiotics. There are several antibiotics that are effective against strep, but it is important to finish the entire course of whichever medication has been prescribed. Remember that you are treating your child to prevent heart damage, so even when she feels better, she needs to finish out the course of antibiotics. It is not necessary in most cases to repeat the throat swab after the antibiotics are finished. If the strepto-coccal bacteria were the cause of the illness, the antibiotics will have taken care of it. A lot of kids are actually "carriers" of the strep bug, meaning that they have it in their throats and pass it around to other kids but don't actually get sick themselves. They will have a positive test *after* taking anti-biotics because the bacteria are happily thriving in there and aren't killed by normal antibiotics. These kids are the little buggers who have a "positive strep test" with a runny nose and cold symptoms. They actually have a cold, but end up receiving unnecessary antibiotics that do absolutely nothing for them. That said, sometimes we will go looking for the little "typhoid" Mary so that we can try to prevent her from making anyone else ill.

If your child does have true strep throat, the most impor-tant things you can do for her are provide ample pain and

## TONSIL REMOVAL

When there is a throat infection (of any kind), the tonsils may become big and inflamed. Previously tonsils were often removed in kids with frequent throat infections, including strep, with the thinking being, no tonsils, no infection. Turns out that isn't entirely true and that you can still get strep throat even after your tonsils are long gone. There are still times when the tonsils should be taken out, but more commonly for kids with tonsils so big they make breathing difficult.

fever control and push the fluids! Her throat really hurts, so Popsicles and ice cream for dinner are fine by me. The antibiotics may decrease (slightly) the time during which a child with strep is contagious, so she should be able to go back to school in twenty-four to forty-eight hours, when the fever is gone and she is feeling well enough to go pick up some other germ from her buddies.

## Mouth and Teeth Injuries

### BLEEDING

Our heads and faces have a rather lavish blood supply compared to the rest of the body, so any injury can cause some pretty impressive bleeding. It usually looks like more blood than it is and should stop within a few moments with some gentle pressure and an end to the crying.

*The Lips and Mouth.* So he fell and bit his lip. Remember that any injury to the face is likely to be quite bloody, so before you panic, apply gentle pressure with a clean cloth to any area of bleeding. Then take a look. A cut on the lip that crosses the border onto the face will require careful suturing to ensure that a good cosmetic outcome is achieved. Call your doc and tell her your kid needs a repair of his *vermillion* border. He'll think you're pompous, but appreciate the detail. Other cuts on the lip usually don't need repair unless they are very large. Cuts on the inside of the lips are often not repaired because they heal so quickly on their own. Repairing such wounds is difficult and increases the risk of infection. For cuts inside the mouth and lips, the most important step in caring for these wounds is keeping them clean. If your baby is small, gently wiping the cut with a damp, clean cloth after feeding is sufficient. For older kids, a good rinse with water after eating should help wash away any food residue that has gotten into the wound.

*Inside the Mouth.* The mouth is a pretty wet place. Wounds along the lips, gums, and inside the mouth aren't going to look the same as elsewhere while they are healing. Think about when you go in a swimming pool with a scab on your knee. After you get out, the scab has turned all mushy and white. Wounds inside the mouth look the same while healing. Don't be alarmed. For all sores inside the mouth, be careful of food or drink that is particularly spicy, salty, or acidic, such as potato chips and orange juice. They will sting! Instead, give your kid as many Popsicles as he wants and rest assured that most cuts inside the mouth heal within two to three days.

*The Tongue.* Kids fall and bite their tongue all the time. It is very difficult to convince parents that the vast majority of tongue wounds require no care whatsoever. Even with large cuts along the side or in the front, very few actually need repair. These wounds will uniformly heal quite nicely without intervention. But no one wants to believe this. So you will find a dentist or doctor who is willing to take the time to restrain your child and struggle to get one or two stitches into his tongue while trying to keep all his fingers. And as soon as he is done, your kid might just bite right through his stitch and spit it out. It's usually not worth the trouble in my book. Cold things, like Popsicles, may also help control the bleeding, as will sitting quietly. The cut will open back up and begin to bleed again if your baby gets excited or upset and this is okay. That said, very large cuts or cuts that are bleeding heavily after ten to fifteen minutes of quiet rest may require intervention. If in doubt, call your pediatrician.

**Teeth and Gums.** If your baby hasn't sprouted any teeth yet and has cut or injured her gums, gentle pressure will stop the bleeding and sucking on something cold will help with the pain. In rare cases, an injury to the gum may cause injury to the developing tooth underneath, but the damage is done. You may want to touch base with the family dentist in the next few days.

Injuries to teeth can be categorized in several ways. The tooth may be knocked loose or slightly moved. In this case, the ligaments and connective tissues holding the tooth in place have been damaged. If the tooth is very loose, it may need to be removed. Otherwise, there is nothing to do except watch and wait. If the root of the tooth has been injured, the

### EMERGENCY!

If your kid knocks out a *baby* tooth, we are never going to reimplant the tooth into the socket. Just get out your wallet and pay the tooth fairy. Adult teeth are another matter. Don't touch the root. Rinse the tooth gently and place it back in the tooth socket of a child old enough not to accidentally swallow it, or into a glass of milk. Truly paranoid parents might want to have a special tooth-saving solution such as Save-a-Tooth in the medicine cupboard. The mouth is not only the best environment for an injured tooth, but the faster the tooth can be put back into the empty socket, the better chance it has to survive. Take the tooth, and the kid attached to the mouth from whence the tooth came, to your dentist, pediatrician, or emergency room as soon as possible. If it seems that the tooth has a chance of survival, the dentist can apply a brace to help stabilize the tooth while it tries to heal.

tooth may turn gray and die or can possibly become infected. In either case, a dentist is best equipped to handle this situation, but not on an emergent basis.

If the tooth has been pushed up into the gums, you may or may not be able to see any of it. This can make it difficult to know if the tooth has broken off or been knocked out. Regardless, there is nothing for you to do right at this moment. Baby teeth are designed to get knocked around when your kid smacks his face against the coffee table. When pushed all the way back into the gum (intruded), the tooth may or may not have damaged the developing adult tooth but there is nothing you can do about it now. The baby tooth will probably come back down into position over time. Whether the tooth survives, or has damaged the new tooth underneath, no one can know. Your dentist or pediatrician may want to see your child within a couple of days to evaluate the condition (and location!) of the intruded tooth, as well as watch for damage to the developing teeth.

With either an intrusion or an avulsion (knocked out), if your child is coughing or having difficulty breathing, and you can't see or find the tooth, it is possible that the little chunk of enamel is now sitting in her lungs. Give your doctor a call because she might need an X-ray to make sure that everything is okay.

***Other Mouth Injuries.*** Kids like to run around while holding sharp objects. Occasionally, a kid will fall, sending the sharp object straight into the back of his throat, causing an injury. Anything that is stuck in the mouth or throat (think hair pick or pencil) and not preventing a child from breathing should be left in place and removed only by a doctor. Severe bleeding should also prompt a call to 911. If (most commonly!) all that happens is that the object has fallen out, there is a small cut in the back of the throat, and your child appears otherwise fine, just give your pediatrician a call. Depending on the circumstance, he may want to see you or he may simply follow your child's condition over the phone. You should be aware that injuries to the back of the throat can rarely cause a serious infection of the space between the throat and the neck bones. A child who has had a recent injury to the mouth or throat and develops a fever and refusal to turn her head needs to be seen urgently.

## 911!

If your child has fallen with something in his mouth and is having trouble breathing or bleeding heavily, call 911. If the object is stuck in the mouth, do *not* pull it out. Call an ambulance. We will remove the offending object after we have made sure that no blood vessels have been injured.

## Blisters and Cold Sores

Many viral infections may cause blisters and sores around the lips, on the gums and tongue, and in the back of the throat. Most of us have been exposed to the herpes virus, often as children. There are two types of herpes virus, with one being quite common and causing cold sores and the other causing sores in the genital region. The second type is the one you are panicking about, but rest assured, most cases of herpes infection are *not* sexually transmitted. Either type of the herpes virus may cause symptoms in either place and both are very contagious. The herpes virus lives in us forever once we have been exposed, but acts up with varying frequency as the virus goes to sleep and then becomes lively again. The first bout of herpes can cause an absolutely miserable illness called herpetic gingivostomatitis, which basically means that the sores are not only on the lips, but also on the gums (gingiva) and tongue (stoma). In addition to terrible sores everywhere, babies and little kids can have very high fevers and the illness can last up to two weeks. If caught very early, there is a prescription medicine that may shorten the duration of the illness, but it truly needs to be started within the first three days to be effective, which is often before a parent understands what is happening. So most kids just have to weather through it. Other than being painful and contagious, these sores are harmless and will go away within about a week.

## THAT STINGS!

If your little one has sores in or around his mouth, anything that is very spicy, salty, or acidic is going to hurt. Things like orange juice, salty chips, or hot salsa will sting and burn. Cold things will feel good. But she needs to keep herself hydrated. Put down that superacidic lemonade (Ouch, that stings!) and get your kid a Popsicle.

There are other types of viral infections that can cause blisters and sores in the mouth, particularly in the back of the throat. The hand, foot, and mouth virus (called Coxsackie) is a common cause of tiny blisters over the back part of the roof of the mouth. There is nothing to do about these sores except have patience.

For all sores in the mouth, pain medicine is good, as are cold things, like Popsicles and ice cream for older babies and kids. The biggest concern we have for kids with viral blisters in their mouth is preventing dehydration, so really try to encourage your baby to keep drinking and provide liberal pain control. Your doctor may also be able to give you suggestions for medication to put directly onto the sores. Be very careful, however, about using over-the-counter products without consulting your doctor.

> ### EMERGENCY!
>
> If your kid has eaten an entire tube of *any* type (adult or infant) of teething or mouth sore medication, call the Poison Center (1-800-222-1222) *immediately*.

## Thrush

Should you notice a white coating over your little one's lips or tongue, well, first try just wiping it off with a damp cloth. If it comes off, it is milk. Stop messing with him. But if the white areas seem thick and you can't wipe them away, that is called thrush. Thrush is a fungal infection that can grow in a baby's mouth, on his pacifier or bottles, and even on your breast. Some babies find this infection painful or irritating, and they may act as if they don't want to eat. Your doctor can provide you with a prescription medication. Because thrush is simply an overgrowth of the fungus that we find growing normally on all of us, it may reappear over time. Be sure to sterilize all pacifiers and bottle nipples as soon as you begin treatment. Remember that fungi like warm, moist places, making a baby's mouth a perfect place to take over and grow inside. (Think other warm, wet places and go read about diaper rashes in Chapter 9.)

## Spots on the Tongue

As I've said, certain viral infections may cause spots and blisters on the tongue. These are painful, but not harmful, and your biggest job is preventing dehydration. Some kids have what is called a geographic tongue, meaning that there are funny patterns and swirls on its surface all the time, not just when he is sick. This is totally normal and may or may not go away with time. And by the way, the bumps on his tongue *are* taste buds, and yes, they are supposed to be that big. Or small. Whatever.

## Teething

Most babies will have a tooth by six months of age, and you should definitely let your doctor know if there aren't any by the age of one. Parents spend a lot of time worrying about teething and the myriad of symptoms for which it is blamed. However, teething gives you teeth. It doesn't cause fever or diarrhea or a runny nose or any of that other stuff. Colds and viruses do, and a lot of kids who are teething happen to have a runny nose. Some people will say that a very low-grade fever can occur when the tooth erupts, yet it is more likely to be a virus to blame than the tooth. But teething can be uncomfortable for some babies. A lot of babies want to chew on something to help relieve the pain, so offering a cool, wet washcloth may help. As with other mouth pain, medicines like acetaminophen may be helpful, as will cold things. Be careful with the frozen teething ring! Babies who suck too frequently on very cold or frozen things may literally freeze the fat cells of their cheeks to death. We call it Popsicle panniculitis, *panniculitis* meaning inflammation of fat cells. Babies with Popsicle panniculitis will develop hard red lumps

## TEETHING GEL

Over-the-counter teething gels are generally safe, but be sure to use a product specifically designed for infants and never more than the recommended dose and frequency. These medications can cause seizures and other problems when given in too high a dose. Also, beware that alcohol (such as in Grandma's whiskey) can be absorbed through the gums and will have a much stronger and potentially dangerous effect on a little one.

on either cheek. This will go away with time and doesn't require any treatment.

## Bad Breath

Most cases of bad breath, or halitosis, can be blamed on little other than borderline hygiene. However, a few conditions may cause a change in the smell of your child's breath. For example, stomach acid that is rising up into the esophagus (reflux) may cause a sour smell. And infections of the throat, such as strep, may cause a change in your kiddo's breath. A foreign body in the nose could make his breath stinky too. A very sweet smell, described as "fruity," can be detected in the breath of someone who is very sick with diabetes, but it is extremely unlikely that your baby would otherwise look well. If in doubt, give your pediatrician a call.

## EMERGENCY!

If your kid has funny, fruity-smelling breath and is having vomiting, difficulty breathing, or is very listless, call your doctor immediately.

# the guts

We really are just one big tube, from mouth to anus. What goes in usually comes out. Sometimes it comes out the wrong way or too fast or slow or thick or thin. Sometimes it creates havoc while inside there. And sometimes kids eat lightbulbs. In this chapter we'll talk about tummyaches and other maladies of the gastrointestinal system, including a fascinating discussion of the colors of poop. Most important, this is where you will find all the information you ever wanted to know about preventing and treating dehydration *at home*, so you might get to skip a trip to the ER.

## Abdominal Pain

### Why Does It Hurt?

"Abdominal pain" is a very common complaint in the ER and one that makes us quietly groan inside. The causes of belly pain in children range from absolutely nothing to potentially life-threatening conditions, and getting to the root of abdominal pain in little kids can be tough. Very simple and nonthreatening conditions may cause a child to scream and writhe, while more serious problems, such as appendicitis, develop over time, meaning that they may initially present with very nonspecific symptoms. That is why for most cases of belly pain, serial phone calls to your pediatrician may be much more useful than running to the emergency room at the first yelp of pain.

> ## MY TUMMY HURTS
>
> When a kid's belly hurts "all over," especially if the pain is crampy or makes him writhe about, it is more likely due to constipation than anything else. Even if he is crying in pain. See if you can get him to toot or poop, maybe by popping him on the potty for a while and getting him to relax by reading a few books or playing a video game.

## Pain from Constipation

The absolute number one cause of belly pain in kids who come to the ER is constipation. I don't care if you tell me he goes every day. There still can be a whole lot of poop up there. Does your kid have "toilet-plugging specials"? Are his stools hard when he goes, or does he leave "skid marks" in his underwear? Even if the answer is "no," a child still may have belly pain because of constipation. Abdominal pain from constipation tends to hurt "all over," is only rarely accompanied by vomiting or fever, and doesn't hurt any more or less when a kid moves, jumps, or rides in a car. A child may scream and writhe and then seem fine a few minutes later, since the pain is intense but comes and goes. If you suspect that your child may be a victim of his own stool, try having him sit on the potty for a while. Your pediatrician may recommend a dose of milk of magnesia or another over-the-counter laxative. Alternatively, some folks really like using rectal suppositories or a pediatric enema. Personally, I prefer the suppositories, since I find the enema to be punitive to both child and parent (and nurse, if in the ER). But if a kid is in dire straits and desperately needs to poop, you do what you've got to do. Of note, do *not* make your own enema at home using water or soap or anything else. You might cause serious injury or illness!

For more on constipation, flip to page 130.

## Intussusception

Another less common, albeit more concerning, cause of belly pain in older babies and toddlers is called intussusception, which means a telescoping of the bowel. In this condition, the bowel slides in on itself, like a telescope, most commonly at the juncture of the large and small intestines. The telescoping intermittently tightens on itself, causing a decrease in blood flow to that part of the intestines, which in turn causes significant pain. Kids with intussusception will be perfectly fine, running around and playing, then suddenly develop intense belly pain that causes them to cry and draw their knees into their bellies. After a minute or so, the pain eases and the kid goes on her merry way, only to have another episode awhile later. Rarely, intussusception may present in a completely opposite manner, with severe, continuous lethargy. In either case, intussusception may be accompanied by true bilious vomiting (green like a Christmas tree, not yellow), although the vomit may look normal in the beginning. Blood may appear in the stools and might look like red jelly, although this doesn't usually happen right away. Diarrhea is rare. The reason we need to make this diagnosis is because with time the telescoped section of the bowel might start to die from a lack of oxygen. If this happens, infection may occur or surgery may be necessary. Therefore, we'd like to diagnose intussusception early. The diagnosis is made when a radiologist pushes air or a special dye into the baby's rectum. If he sees the abnormal bowel, he will continue the procedure until the bowel pops back open. Some radiologists will prefer to perform an ultrasound of the belly to find the intussusception first, hoping to avoid the whole tube up the bum thing. However your hospital handles these cases is a matter of local practice. Remember that in either case, we are trying to prevent serious consequences for your child. If you think your kid may have an intussusception, call your pediatrician immediately.

## COULD IT BE INTUSSUSCEPTION?

Intussusception, or telescoping of the bowel, is most common in kids between three and twelve months old, with the majority of cases being diagnosed in children less than two. However, it can happen to kids of all ages, so don't rule it out if your kid is older or younger.

## Appendicitis

The appendix is a little tail that hangs off the beginning part of the large intestines. Sometimes the appendix can become blocked off and then infected. In the beginning, the pain is usually around the belly button. Vomiting and a fever may also be present. As the inflammation increases, the pain settles into the lower right part of the belly and causes inflammation of the lining of the abdomen, which is called peritonitis. "Peritoneal" abdominal pain is a clue to us that something of significance is happening in there that needs further investigation. Peritonitis causes pain with movement, such as walking, jumping, or riding in the car, and severe pain when touching the belly, which worsens as you let go. If your kid can jump up and down without making the pain worse, it's far less likely to be serious. As the illness progresses, the appendix can rupture, or burst, spreading infected material all over the belly. Early appendicitis is very nonspecific and little ones aren't good at explaining their symptoms. Therefore, in nearly 100 percent of babies and young children with appendicitis, the diagnosis is not made until the appendix has already ruptured.

## Is It Appendicitis?

Not all pain on the right side of the belly is from an inflamed appendix. In fact, it is more likely that he is constipated. Call your doctor if your kid has belly pain, but don't be surprised if she doesn't send you straight to the ER or to her office. Appendicitis isn't only about the location of the pain; it's part of a whole story.

Appendicitis can be very difficult to diagnose in anyone, but children are extra difficult. The only 100 percent test for appendicitis is an operation. Ultrasound or CT scan may be useful studies, but can be both less reliable and more difficult to interpret in children. Blood tests may be normal or abnormal. The most helpful test of all is the test of time, with repeated exams of the belly. Regrettably, we don't always have that luxury in the ER and it is sometimes necessary to have a child seen the next morning again, by either us or by her regular doctor. In other words, if you are worried about appendicitis in your child, call your doctor. Depending on how long she has been sick and what other symptoms are present, you may be sent to the ER or be asked simply to observe your child for a few more hours at home and update your doctor with a few more phone calls.

All in all, belly pain has many, many causes in babies and

children. Infections elsewhere in the body, such as pneumonia, may cause abdominal pain as their primary symptom. Childhood migraines can present as belly pain and vomiting. Strep throat may cause a tummyache. Even stress or tension can cause belly pain, a very common finding in school-age kids. A huge number of older kids have "nonorganic" abdominal pain, meaning there is no detectable medical cause; stress, depression, or problems at school can cause real physical belly pain. This is a horridly frustrating thing for a parent to hear, and a lot of parents get really mad at the doctor who suggests this but it's the truth.

So, if your child is having severe pain, is vomiting dark green, or has a belly that seems bigger, harder, or very tender to you, call your doctor immediately. But remember, no matter what kinds of studies and tests we might order, we may never know the reason for abdominal pain in a fair number of children. In the absence of other signs such as unexplained weight loss, growth failure, or fever, a child who gets seen for belly pain and checks out fine probably is fine. But parents don't like to hear this. And this is why a chief complaint of "abdominal pain" makes us cry a little inside.

## Vomiting

Vomiting with diarrhea is uniformly infectious in nature and we worry mostly about keeping a kid hydrated and making sure that she weathers the storm without complication. When vomiting occurs alone, however, there are many diagnoses to consider. While most causes of vomiting are absolutely nothing to worry about, others are cause for concern. Fortunately, there are a few clues to help us sort out what is what.

First, do not panic at the first vomit. Get a mop. Clean it

up. Put your kid in the tub. Relax. Most cases of a stomach bug, or gastroenteritis, begin with vomiting and the diarrhea occurs later. Most kids with gastroenteritis will vomit repeatedly for several hours and then quiet down a bit, giving you a chance to get some fluids into them. Do *not* panic that your child will become dehydrated within a matter of a few hours. He goes several hours or even all night without food normally, so puking for six hours is not going to get him into trouble.

## WHEN TO CALL THE DOCTOR AND WHEN *NOT* TO

You have my permission to wake your kid's pediatrician if: she vomits dark green, has *repeated* episodes of bloody vomit, is having trouble breathing, or is acting very ill. I'll also let you call if she has severe continuous belly pain, or a belly that is firm or hard, red, seems to be sticking out, or is very tender. Do *not* wake your child's doctor to tell him: the vomit came out the nose or shot across the room, it had bloody streaks in it, it is yellow in color, or because the kid threw up in his sleep.

## Vomiting Blood

Remember that the most common cause of bloody vomit in children is blood coming from somewhere up above, most commonly the nose. So a bit of blood in the vomit is not a cause for panic. A child who has vomited forcefully may also cause little tears in the stomach muscles and have tinges of blood in her vomit. This too is okay. Bleeding of the esophagus, stomach, or intestines can be worrisome but is, fortunately, extremely rare in children. In these patients, the bloody vomit would be recurrent. Repeated episodes of vomiting blood, or vomiting very large amounts of blood or blood clots, should prompt a phone call to your doctor.

## Vomiting Colors

I honestly could care less what color the vomit is until you tell me it is green. And not the yellow-green that comes up when there is nothing left to vomit. That is stomach juice. We are talking green, green, green. Green like a Christmas tree green. Green like my scrub pants green. Bile is the juice produced by our liver that sits in our small intestines waiting to help digest our food. Vomiting true bile means that the vomit is coming from somewhere south of the stomach. Parents always think that bile is yellow, but it isn't. The yellow fluid a kid throws up comes from his tummy when there is nothing left down there but stomach juice. Bile is green, not yellow. While this can rarely occur in patients who are vomiting forcefully or repeatedly, we need to make sure that another problem, such as a twisted intestine or bowel blockage, hasn't happened. Go ahead and call.

## Vomiting Every Day

The stomach is actually a big muscle, as are the valves at the top and bottom, designed to keep food down and allow it to pass through to the rest of the gut. In a baby, these muscles are immature and occasionally get confused. Rather than acting in a coordinated manner to propel food south, sometimes they get a little overexcited, or all squeeze together at once, sending milk back up the esophagus and out the mouth. The valve at the top of the stomach that prevents food from going back north isn't terribly effective either in small babies, but gets tougher and better with time. So most babies will have relatively frequent episodes of "spitting up." In fact, the majority of infants three to four months old will vomit at least once a day. If the vomiting is forceful, the spit-ups may shoot across the room or actually come out his nose. Vomit that shoots out the nose is okay. The mouth is connected to the nose, and vomit will take any available escape route. He will not choke on his vomit. The only people who choke on their vomit are people with an abnormal gag reflex. A normal child who is not stumbling drunk or high on Grandma's sleeping pills will *not* choke on his vomit. Vomit that shoots across the room also seems to frighten people. If it happens only rarely, and your little one is otherwise happy and growing, it's not a problem. Of course, if she is a major chunk and sucking down eight ounces every three hours and spitting up, she's being overfed and you should try to decrease the amount of each feeding while increasing the frequency.

## ARE HER EYES *REALLY* BIGGER?

On the first day of life, a baby's stomach is able to hold just a little over a teaspoon and is about the size of a marble. By Day 3, it can still only hold less than an ounce. As she grows, so will her tummy, always approximating the size of her fist. Hold up her hand and see if you think it can *really* hold eight ounces of formula without consequence.

You may have heard the term *reflux*, which is short for gastroesophageal reflux, where the stomach contents regurgitate into the esophagus. This is considered abnormal in adults and older children and, if it happens, may cause significant heartburn, scarring of the esophagus, and even swelling and irritation of the vocal cords. However, in most babies, it is to be expected because the muscles and valves of the stomach that control the flow of food are weak and floppy and milk can shoot around in any direction. That said, in a few babies and little kids, reflux causes wheezing and coughing or difficulty gaining weight. Whenever there are symptoms other than spitting or vomiting, we call it gastroesophageal reflux disease, which is different from just reflux. In babies, reflux is most often a perfectly normal thing. Your pediatrician can help you decide when a spitty baby has become a problem and together you can determine the best course of action to help your little one along until she grows up a bit.

## THE VOLUME OF VOMIT

Every parent thinks that every vomit is "the whole bottle!" It isn't. Take a bottle and pour it on the floor. I'm serious. Dump four ounces on the linoleum. You'll be surprised. You just think it is the whole bottle because it soaked your shirt and ruined your couch.

As for whether reflux can cause excessive fussiness and crying, most doctors agree that excessive crying in young babies is more likely due to colic than to any medical condition. The short version is that most experts agree that excessive crying in small babies is due to an immature brain. Of course, there is nothing you can do about that except wait for his brain to grow up. Unexplained crying in a baby is so very frustrating and can make parents feel like complete failures, so naturally a tangible explanation and solution are desired. Some babies are put on medications for reflux and heartburn to treat crying. Unfortunately, all too often the answer is that they are just criers.

One condition that deserves mention is pyloric stenosis. Occasionally the muscle that lets food out of the stomach and into the small intestine (the pylorus) will become very thick, preventing this forward passage of stomach contents. This condition tends to run in families and has a tendency to strike firstborn males, but no baby is immune. As this muscle thickens, a baby will begin to vomit with greater frequency and force. Eventually the vomiting is after every single feed and the baby acts ferociously hungry right afterward. Usually by five to six weeks of age, although it can present in babies as young as two weeks, the vomiting will be so frequent that the baby will begin to lose weight or show signs of dehydration. This condition requires a very simple little operation to loosen that muscle and most babies do great and are home in a couple of days. If you are worried that the amount of vomiting the baby is doing is crossing the line from normal to not, first try giving her smaller amounts more frequently. If the vomiting continues, call your pediatrician, who will decide if an ultrasound test is necessary. This test may be difficult for us to get on an emergent basis or in the middle of the night, so as long as the baby is not showing signs of dehydration, the diagnosis can wait for regular business hours.

### WHEN VOMITING DAILY IS A PROBLEM

If your baby vomits every day, fine. But if he is losing weight, becoming dehydrated, or develops breathing troubles, such as wheezing or pneumonia, because of it, that's not normal.

All in all, there are a multitude of perfectly reasonable causes of vomiting in babies and children. On the other hand, problems with the structure of the stomach or intestines, blockages, and certain infections, such as appendicitis, pneumonia, or a kidney infection, may cause vomiting. If your child appears to be in a lot of pain, or his belly seems harder or looks like it is sticking out farther than usual, call your pediatrician.

Vomiting true green or large amounts of blood should also warrant a phone call. Vomiting that occurs in a child with a fever who seems to be very irritable or fussy, or when accompanied by a cough or rapid breathing, also needs to be evaluated. And as always, if you feel your child looks or acts like something is truly wrong, don't hesitate to get your doctor on the line.

## Vomiting and Diarrhea

Vomiting and diarrhea together is called gastroenteritis, meaning infection of the gastrointestinal (stomach and bowels) system. Gastroenteritis is most commonly caused by viral infections. Kids get gastroenteritis all the time, because they touch people and surfaces, pick up germs, and then put their fingers into their little mouths and the mouths of their little buddies. The infections that cause gastroenteritis are passed in what we call a fecal-oral manner. I will spare you the details. I think you get it. Disgusting, eh? Unfortunately, the viruses that cause gastroenteritis are extremely contagious, which means that if one kid gets it, everyone gets it. All you can hope for is that if you are religious about washing your hands and your child's hands, maybe you stand a chance.

Because there are different causes of gastroenteritis, kids may have different symptoms at different times. Some viruses cause a horribly watery, profuse diarrhea. Some cause the most foul-smelling diarrhea. Others may give you more vomiting and less diarrhea, and so on. In addition, some infections, particularly bacterial ones, may cause bloody diarrhea. In cases of bloody diarrhea, your doctor will want to culture the stool to determine which, if any, type of bacteria is causing the infection. We don't treat a suspected case of bacterial gastroenteritis with antibiotics until we know exactly what is causing the illness. Antibiotics may make a child with certain infections much sicker or can increase the risk that a child will become a "carrier," meaning that he is no longer sick but delightfully passes his germs along to others. So do *not* reach into the cupboard and get out the leftover antibiotics that you've been hoarding. There are times when antibiotic therapy is absolutely necessary for patients with a bacterial infection of the gut, but they are less common than you might imagine, and your doctor knows when it is the right time to treat one and when it is better to let it run its course.

## Your Menagerie

Owning pets can increase the risk that a child has a *bacterial* cause of his vomiting and diarrhea, although the vast majority will still just have a virus. *But* if you've got pets, particularly reptiles of any kind, mention it when you call your doctor.

Other than worrying about dehydration, there is little for us to say or do about vomiting and diarrhea. Most cases will get better within three to five days, although the symptoms may continue for a few more. Along with ensuring that your little one is getting enough fluid, getting her back to her regular diet as soon as possible will actually help speed her recovery. However, the bowels may still need a little time to recuperate and the diarrhea may continue for up to a couple of weeks after the infection has resolved. Withholding certain foods, such as dairy, is not recommended for most kids. The intestines will recover faster when given a regular diet. In rare cases, a child may have trouble digesting certain foods, such as the main sugar found in dairy products (lactose), for a period of time. If your child is recovering from gastroenteritis and seems to develop pain and diarrhea, or is exceptionally gassy after drinking cow's milk, speak to your pediatrician. For a very small number of children, a temporary ban on dairy products may be helpful, but for the vast majority of children, returning to their regular diet as soon as possible is the best treatment.

## Dehydration

When a child develops vomiting or diarrhea, or both, her hydration status is on everyone's mind. Dehydration means that the body has less fluid than normal, which can make the heart beat faster, cause less-frequent urination, or turn a kid into a listless lump. With very mild dehydration, very few signs may be apparent. As the dehydration worsens, a drop in urine production occurs, as well as a drying out of the mouth and eyes. With severe dehydration, a child is extremely listless, with a sunken soft spot, a dry, cracked tongue, and skin that doesn't snap back into place when pinched. The good news is that almost all cases of dehydration can be prevented, and cases of mild to moderate dehydration can be managed at home, without IV fluids or fancy equipment. If, however, despite your best efforts, your tyke is developing worsening dehydration, you should call your pediatrician, who can help you decide if this is something that can wait until morning or needs to be seen more urgently. Signs of moderate dehydration include a dry tongue and mouth, no tears when crying, and a pretty noticeable decrease in activity and energy. I don't worry so much about her lips, since mine are dry and cracked no matter what my hydration status is, and crying tears is a toughie, since some kids are better at it than others. The number of wet diapers that little Beauregard is producing is not a terribly reliable screening method for dehydration. These fancy modern diapers are so absorbent, it can be really difficult to find the urine. Plus if she's got diarrhea, the urine is all mixed in there and you can't tell the difference. In general, diagnosing a child with dehydration means taking a look at the whole kid.

## Is She Dehydrated?

A child who is happy and smiley is not dehydrated, no matter how little fluid you think she's had that day. No matter how many wet diapers. I promise.

Ideally, you want to prevent your child from becoming dehydrated in the first place. When she is sick, offer liberal amounts of fluids, of any kind that she wants. Specific rehydration products, such as Pedialyte or Ricelyte, are designed for the *treatment* of dehydration, not its prevention. They aren't magic formulas that will keep the evil spirits away. The ideal food and drink to prevent dehydration is your child's regular diet. If he is on breast milk or formula, continue feeding as usual, although you may need to offer smaller, more frequent amounts if his tummy is upset. For older babies and children, Popsicles, milk, water, and juice are fine, although be aware that very sugary juices and sodas will cause a worsening of the diarrhea, as sugar pulls water into the intestines. Fruit juices such as apple, pear, and prune are particularly offensive, which is why we use them to treat *constipation*. If your kid is absolutely insistent on his fruit juice, try watering it down. Bubbly water might make it a bit more "special."

If, despite your full-on fluid assault, your little one begins to exhibit signs of dehydration, do *not* panic. You can probably manage this at home. While many parents have bought into the belief that only IV fluids can treat dehydration, study after study has shown that rehydrating a child by *mouth*, or oral rehydration, is actually superior to IV fluids, even when performed in the emergency room. The first and most obvious reason is how much time, money, and effort can be saved. Second, the child is spared the discomfort of what may be several attempts at an IV, since a vein is more difficult to locate in a dehydrated child, or in a chubby one for that matter, as well as any possible complications from being stuck with a needle, such as local inflammation at the IV site. And third, a child will actually *recover faster* when given oral rehydration as opposed to IV fluids. Why then, you ask, do so many kids get IV fluids to treat dehydration when they come to the ER? One reason is that we have been beaten into submission by the parade of exhausted and frustrated parents insisting that oral rehydration can't *possibly* work. Second, proper oral rehydration requires good instruction and is time-intensive.

Oral rehydration is an actual procedure, with a measuring cup and a stopwatch. Remember that *rehydration* is different from preventing dehydration. Now is the time to grab a solution that is specifically designed for restoring fluid to the body. These products work by combining salt with sugar, which helps your intestines absorb fluid in a different way. Since your child's gut is bruised and battered from fighting the infection, this alternative system helps maximize fluid uptake. Whether you are using a powder that is mixed with water (the WHO electrolyte solution), or a commercial product such as Pedialyte or Ricelyte, make sure that it is appropriate for infants and children. Sports drinks such as Gatorade are too high in sugar and too concentrated to treat dehydration in babies and little kids. Juices, water, and soda do not have the appropriate amounts of salt and other electrolytes that are essential for replacing fluid in a dehydrated child. Of course, if a little squirt of her favorite juice mixed into the rehydration solution will increase her willingness to drink it, go ahead. But just a little squirt.

Once you have gathered your materials, here is how it is going to work: controlled small amounts at preset time intervals. If you successfully make it to one hour, you can double the amount the next hour, gradually increasing the volume of fluid until your child is rehydrated or able to drink freely. If she vomits, wait thirty minutes and then start over.

## THE REHYDRATION PROCEDURE

1 teaspoon, or 5 milliliters (ml), for babies and little kids (up to about four or five years old) every five minutes for one hour. You can get a medication syringe from most pharmacies. Kids older than four or five who can handle a little more fluid can start at 2 teaspoons, or 10 ml. Then double it for the next hour. Do *not* give her more. She *will* throw it back up.

Once you begin the process of oral rehydration, you will quickly realize that 1 teaspoon is a very small amount of fluid. Since your poor peanut is dehydrated, she is thirsty, and is going to cry and act pathetic. Do *not* give in. The tiny bit that goes into the tummy won't be large enough to upset an already tenuous situation. And the tiny amount of fluid will partly be absorbed before it can be vomited back out. If you cave and hand over the whole bottle, the large volume of liquid that she sucks down will come right back up. Easy does it.

If your child vomits occasionally but is gradually becoming perkier, you are doing great. Remember that a fair amount of fluid has already been absorbed before she had a chance to vomit again. As for when you can stop, most kids will be much improved after two hours of oral rehydration. The exact amount of fluid a dehydrated child needs can be estimated but I'm not going to tell you how. That will make you crazy. Know that in the first two hours of oral rehydration, you have replaced enough fluid that she should be able to drink the rest of whatever she needs by herself over the next several hours. You've hydrated her gently, helping to restore her blood sugar and rinse away the starvation hormones, both of which worsen nausea and vomiting. So her vomiting will improve as her hydration status gets better. Good job!

## Gas

Here is the classic "chicken or egg" question for all of us. Do you cry because you have gas, or is it possible that you have gas because you are crying? Many of us now believe that an irritable, crying infant is not crying because his belly hurts. All babies turn red and purple when they cry, and they all draw their legs up and tighten up their belly muscles. A baby's body is far softer and more collapsible than that of a grown-up. Therefore, babies tend to use a lot more muscles when moving their chest walls, such as when they cry, or even breathe. But this also means that when your kid really wants to let you have it, he's going to use every muscle at his disposal and make himself heard. Turning colors, tensing up, or turning red before passing gas are normal baby behaviors. "Gas drops" and other over-the-counter products designed to treat these "symptoms" are generally not harmful, but they also aren't helpful and are probably a waste of money. So, if I was a baby and somebody gave me some "gas drops" to help my tummy and they tasted disgusting and made me cry and then I accidentally swallowed more air because I'm, after all, just a baby, and then I got a tummyache because I was full of gas, I'd be pretty annoyed. To reiterate, simethicone, the main ingredient in most "gas drops," has never been shown to be any more effective for infant gas or crying than hen's teeth or fairy dust. Medicines that don't do anything even when people swear by them are called placebos.

If you are worried because your baby seems to pass a lot of gas, particularly if it happens in embarrassing situations and is noticeably foul smelling, this is completely normal. Honestly, what did you expect? Roses?

## All Things Poop

### Constipation

Many parents come to the ER to report that the baby has not produced stool in a socially acceptable time frame. Remember that all babies are as different as their poop. If he is breastfed and hasn't started cereal or solids, think creamed corn. However, some babies, especially those who are formula fed, will produce stools that look like anything from canned vegetables to normal adult formed stool. The consistency and color are of less interest to us than you might think. Also, some babies poop five times a day; some poop once a week. If you poop once a week and it is soft, that is not constipation. I'm unexcited.

Constipation means that the stools that come out are hard, rocklike, and difficult to pass. A baby is not necessarily "constipated" when he doesn't create stool on demand. All babies turn red and grunt and draw their legs up when they poop. If you were too dumb to know that you have to relax your little butt muscles *and* you were lying on your back trying to stool in *your* pants, you would also likely turn red and make some funny noises. Of course, I know that your baby is a genius. But there is still a learning curve here. Babies have to learn to relax their anus and to use their stomach muscles to push the poop out. Learning how to push and squeeze makes babies wiggle and squirm. For a baby that is truly constipated, some physicians advocate a daily ounce of water, some an ounce of sugar water, some an ounce of watered-down prune or pear juice. However, most babies are not actually constipated, and patience is all that is necessary. If your baby actually is constipated, your doctor can help you decide on a course of action. There is no rush here. As long as your baby is happy, has a nice soft belly, is eating, and is passing gas, no worries. Do not panic. Don't try to stick anything in there to "stimulate a poop." Do *not* try to pull the poop out with a Q-tip.

## Is It Constipation?

All babies turn red and grunt when pooping. Constipation is hard stool. A baby who produces soft stool once a week, and is otherwise happy and well, is not constipated and doesn't need any treatment. School-age kids, however, who poop once a week might actually have a problem and may develop encopresis. Keep reading.

Older toddlers and young children may develop constipation for several reasons. A change in diet, a recent illness, or a change in routine may cause a temporary bout of constipation. Potty training is another stressor that can make a kid constipated. Little boys, in particular, seem to fall victim to this. Maybe because some of them see a sticklike object fall into the toilet and get flushed away into obscurity, and then they get nervous about other things that might fall off and be lost forever. I don't know. I'm just free-associating here. Some kids are too busy to go to the potty or can't be bothered to sit there long enough. Whether it is impatience, fear, resistance to change, or the power struggles that can come with potty training, a voluntary withholding of stools can lead to a more severe form of constipation called encopresis, which is a relatively common condition in school-age kids, who don't want to stop playing to come inside and have a poop. With encopresis, the buildup of stool causes a stretching of the bowel. The brain eventually gets tired of the constant signals being sent from the stretch sensors of the intestines and stops listening. So the child loses the urge to have a bowel movement. With time, the backup of stool increases, with increasing stretching of the bowel, until liquid stool from above begins to leak around the big poo ball. This leakage is impossible to control and results in "skid marks" or stool stains in the underwear.

If your toddler or child has developed constipation only recently, make sure that he is getting plenty of fluids. You can also try to increase the fiber in his diet. Try sprinkling a little bran cereal on his Frosted Flakes. Honestly, there are some mighty tasty bran cereals out there that make great snacks. Encourage fruits and vegetables. Alternatively, a nighttime tablespoon of milk of magnesia or some Maalox should do the trick. (Try stirring it into some ice cream.) Be aware that some of the children's formulations of these medications may be purposely designed *not* to loosen stools, so ask your pediatrician if you aren't sure. Or if you prefer, there are a multitude

## FOODS THAT MAKE YOU POOP

Try offering your kid natural laxatives like the foods that start with *p*: peaches, plums, prunes, pears, peas, and the like. Think *p* for *poop*. Bananas and applesauce don't start with *p*, do they? Those two are better for treating diarrhea!

of gentle over-the-counter laxative products for children, such as senna, that are mild enough and perfectly safe for occasional usage.

## POTTY TRAINING

If you think that potty training is the reason for sudden constipation, it is okay to put the project on hold for a couple of months. Maybe he's just not ready. It's not worth the both of you getting upset and angry.

For kids with more chronic constipation, including those who have gone so far as to develop encopresis, a more multifaceted approach is necessary. Not only will you have to get all the old poop out (often with laxatives or enemas), but also the newly forming stools must be kept soft. Ideally, everything should be so nice and lubricated that he can't resist going to the bathroom. At the same time, it is important to have him sit on the potty at regular intervals, not just when he has the urge to go, because his brain won't recognize the signals. Every day after meals is a good time, because a full belly sends a message to our brains to let the poop come out. Remember Grandpa after Thanksgiving dinner? Honestly, it's called the gastrocolic reflex. Have him sit on the toilet long enough to play an entire video game or read a couple of books. A system of rewards and prizes may be helpful, such as a star chart tacked to the fridge. Sitting on the potty and pooping every day gets you a prize, like maybe a trip to the park. Remember to be positive, because getting mad or punishing him will only make the situation worse. Treating chronic constipation and encopresis in kids is a long road, and it is very important that you speak with your pediatrician to create a long-term plan.

If despite all your best efforts, your child is unable to produce any stool, and is increasingly uncomfortable, call your pediatrician. Constipation can cause really impressive belly pain in kids that can come and go and cause a lot of yelling and misery. If your child is potty trained, you may have no idea how often he is having a bowel movement or whether the stools are hard or soft. Asking him won't get you a reliable answer.

If your baby has always (since birth) produced very infrequent or very thin and ribbonlike stool, please let your doctor know. These may be signs of a condition where the bowel is very narrow and doesn't move in waves like it should. This is called Hirschsprung's disease and requires an operation to remove the abnormal section of the bowel. This condition is pretty rare, and these kids often have trouble gaining weight and are small. So if he's in hefty-sized pants, it's probably the processed food causing the troubles and not a serious medical condition, but if in doubt, ask your doctor.

## Poop Colors

What about the color? Yellow, green, orange, brown, I don't really care.

*White:* Call your pediatrician. Completely white stools may signify a very rare liver problem in babies.
*Black:* Read "Blood in the Poop," below, but you should know that several foods can cause black, tarry stools, so before you panic, examine your kid's diet. Has your baby suddenly discovered Oreos? That will do it. Black licorice and blueberries too. Of course, I *know* that you didn't give your baby adult Pepto-Bismol (it contains an aspirinlike medication and is *not* for children) or a nice,

cold Guinness, so I don't have to mention those. But other medications, such as iron supplements, may cause very dark stools.

*Red:* Again, see below, but think diet once more. Red Pedialyte, Kool-Aid, Gatorade, or fruit juice can do this. Think red Popsicles, red candy. Basically anything that has red coloring as an additive. By the way, there is a rather popular antibiotic by the name of cefdinir (Omnicef) that tastes like a fabulous bowl of strawberries but will come out bright red in the poop.

*Purple or blue:* That, my friends, is food coloring. Shame on you.

## Blood in the Poop

Blood in the stools certainly sounds alarming, but in kids, it is rarely that worrisome. Most commonly, a stool (usually big and hard) will have bright red streaks of blood along the outside. This is the result of the large, difficult-to-pass stool creating tiny tears in the rectum on its way out. Not to worry and nothing to do, other than to address the underlying constipation. You can put a little petroleum jelly down there to make the poop slide out more easily if you are really worried. If the stool is actually loose, with strings of blood and mucus mixed throughout, this is truly bloody stool and requires evaluation. The most common cause of bloody stool in a baby is allergic colitis, which may occur in young babies, even up to the age of six months. In this case, the baby has developed sensitivity to something in his diet, the most common offending agents being cow's milk and soy proteins. Breastfed babies are not immune, however, and may become sensitized to something in Mom's diet. In this case, a call to the pediatrician is warranted. Dietary adjustments, such as changing

Mom's diet or switching to a specialized hypoallergenic formula, will often resolve the issue, although there may still be some blood in the stools for up to a couple of weeks as his poor little irritated GI tract heals. Notably, these babies are generally happy and growing well and not at all bothered by their condition.

Another cause of truly bloody stool in a baby can be an infection, which has caused irritation and bleeding of the intestines, as discussed in "Vomiting and Diarrhea," on page 123. Bloody diarrhea should prompt a call to your doctor. But as long as your baby looks otherwise pretty happy and content, has a nice soft belly, and is drinking well, it can wait until morning.

An infant who is passing large amounts of blood in his stool, or who passes anything resembling bloody gelatin or "currant jelly," should be evaluated immediately. "Currant jelly" is how we describe the classic very bloody stool, but nobody knows what that is anymore. Think a really dark red grape jelly. Frank blood in place of stool should also prompt a quick evaluation. In addition, bloody stools in the presence of irritability, vomiting, significant pain, or a belly that looks bigger or feels harder than normal should also be urgently evaluated.

### Worms in the Poop

If your kid poops a worm, don't panic. Put it in a container and take it to your pediatrician the next day. She may want to have it identified depending on how your kid is otherwise or if you've been doing something weird like drinking river water while traveling through a jungle. Most kids will just get a short course of medication that will kill any remaining parasites.

## Swallowed Foreign Bodies

I once took care of a toddler who decided to take a huge bite out of a cluster of minilightbulbs. She did it right in front of her mother. Bold. Whether on purpose or by accident, curious little kids will sometimes eat things that aren't food. Money seems to be pretty popular. Quarters in particular. So what do you do if you suspect, or witness, your baby swallowing something that is not generally considered a food source?

### SHE ATE A BOWL OF ROCKS

If your kid eats something that is not normally considered edible (but isn't possibly poisonous), like money, rocks, buttons, hair barrettes, yarn, or marbles, and is acting fine, doesn't have trouble breathing, and is able to eat and drink normally, she's fine. Magnets and disc batteries are a problem and you need to call your doctor. If you aren't sure whether your kid ate something that is potentially dangerous or not, call the Poison Center: 1-800-222-1222.

If your kid is coughing, gagging, or having trouble breathing, go ahead and call an ambulance. Foreign objects can go down the wrong tube into the lungs and this is an emergency. Occasionally an object, such as a quarter or half-dollar, will go down the right tube but become stuck on its way to the stomach. When this happens, it usually is stuck for good, and will have to be removed in the operating room by a specialist. If you suspect that there may be a foreign body stuck somewhere above the stomach, because she is consistently drooling or refusing to eat or drink, or is vomiting every time she tries to take something down, don't give her anything else to eat or drink until you have called your doctor.

If she seems totally fine, you still need to call your doctor, but you can relax. Most of the time, we will still want to have a kid seen pretty soon, so that we can be sure that the object has reached the stomach. Sometimes a doctor will use either an X-ray or a metal detector; other times we will just look at a child. If the object she swallowed isn't something that will show up on X-ray (like a plastic toy), we are forced to rely on nothing more than the kid's behavior to reassure us that all is well.

As noted above, there are certain foreign objects that children swallow that will require immediate evaluation. Disc batteries are an example. A disc battery may become stuck on its way to the stomach and a child may have no symptoms. However, the battery fluid will cause serious damage if it begins to leak, and may even be life threatening. If we have an X-ray showing the battery to be in the stomach, we will just follow up with you in a few days. If it is in the esophagus, however, immediate removal in the operating room is required. Magnets are also in the category of things we want to know about, especially if there are more than one. Two or more magnets may stick together when they get to the intestines, causing serious damage to the bowel tissue caught between them. And last, if a child has swallowed anything that is too long to make it round all the bends in the intestines (e.g., a toothbrush) or has very sharp edges (e.g., a razor or safety pin), we want to see him. Very sharp objects, such as nails and safety pins, usually get coated in mucus and goop and pass through just fine, but occasionally need to be removed.

As for combing through her poop looking for the object, you don't have to do this unless it's an object of value. Repeat X-rays to make sure the offending object has come out the other end are not routinely recommended. If your kid seems to be acting fine, eating normally, and having regular bowel movements, you can pretty much assume everything is fine.

> **WARNING!**
>
> If your little one develops episodes of vomiting or belly pain after ingesting a foreign body, has a belly that feels very hard or is sticking out more and she is uncomfortable, or has blood in her poop, she needs to be seen immediately. These would be very rare occurrences after swallowing most commonly ingested foreign bodies, such as coins, and may be totally unrelated to the foreign object, but still necessitate a call to your doctor.

## Abdominal Trauma

Kids fall down. They jump off furniture. Sometimes they take a hit to the belly. If one of your children gets angry and kicks the other in the stomach, or if your kid hits the side of the trampoline as he tumbles to the ground, pay attention if he says his belly hurts. In the absence of violent injury, such as a car accident, injury to the abdominal organs and intestines is rare, but can happen. Significant bruising of the skin over the abdomen should warrant a phone call to your doctor, as should severe pain, a firm or tense belly, dark green or bloody vomit, or blood in the urine or stool. A classic belly injury in kids occurs when a child crashes his bike and takes the handlebars in the stomach. A strong blow to the belly can cause bleeding and bruising of the intestines, which might result in swelling and a blockage. So, if your child isn't acting right, or you are in any way concerned, call your pediatrician.

# the plumbing

I think this chapter is pretty obvious. Everybody is obsessed with what is happening in the kid's diaper. Is he peeing enough? Should it be that color? Is his hoohah supposed to look like that? Where did her vagina go? You are not alone; these are the questions every parent asks. Let's talk about everything having to do with the kidney and bladder, the manufacturing of urine, and the care and maintenance of the parts that determine whether the cigars are pink or blue.

## Tinkle Tinkle Little Star

### Urine Output

Infants wet their diapers between six and thirty times a day. Well, that is quite a range. How do you know if your sweet pea is generating enough urine? There are lots of reasons why a baby may be making more or less urine than normal. If you think little Hans is outside the range of normal, mention this to your physician.

Many parents may think their baby isn't making enough urine and come to the ER worried about dehydration. And when I get in the room, the kid is smiling, laughing, drooling, drinking, and basically dripping wet. As I've mentioned, today's commercial diapers sometimes make finding the urine a challenge. They are true engineering wonders, are super-absorbent and leakproof. Handy at a family picnic, not so help-ful when you're worried about the baby. If you are worried that your babe isn't peeing, try tucking a small piece of tissue or some cotton balls onto the part of the diaper where your little one is most likely to aim a stream of urine (middle for girls, front for boys). This allows you to know definitively whether or not Marge has successfully produced urine.

Another thing to keep in mind if your kid has diarrhea: Diarrhea can be very watery and run all over the diaper, making it impossible to know if there is any urine mixed into the mess. Of course, diarrhea can cause dehydration, which makes parents very concerned about the frequency of wet diapers. Fortunately, there are other signs and symptoms of dehydration that we can look out for, so go check out "Dehydration," on page 125.

## Ooh, What's That Smell?!

Smelly pee. In medical school, we had to memorize a long list of different pee smells and the diseases with which they are associated. Stinky feet pee. Burnt sugar pee. But if little Arlene's pee smells funny, don't panic. These diseases are extremely rare. It is more likely that she got into some aspara-gus. Seriously, though, any funny odor in your baby's urine should be mentioned to your doctor. Urine that becomes cloudy or smelly probably doesn't mean anything but still should be checked out, especially if she has a fever or is other-wise ill. Depending on how sick she is, this probably can wait until morning, but call your doctor and double-check.

## Is That Blood in His Pee?

If you think he's peed blood, don't panic. First, if the "blood" is actually more pinkish orange, it's not blood at all.

We all have something called uric acid in our urine. Some-times this substance forms little crystals in the diaper, which are commonly mistaken for blood. It means nothing.

Other times there really will be blood in the urine. A bit of blood can point to an infection in the urine or some other kidney or bladder abnormality. While this needs to be inves-tigated, it's not immediately life threatening. Your doctor can perform a simple urine test to confirm that there is actu-ally blood in the urine and to help guide the next step of the evaluation.

## It Burns!

If you've ever had a bladder infection, then you know how it feels. In doctor-talk, an infection in the urine is called a UTI (urinary tract infection). A urine infection can cause a kid to go more frequently and have discolored or bloody urine or abdominal pain. A UTI may also cause burning or pain (dysuria) with urination, so bad she simply refuses to uri-nate because of the pain. UTIs are much more common in little girls than in boys, although some boys, particularly those with abnormalities of the structure of their plumbing, may be more prone to an infection. Any situation in which bacteria enter the normally sterile bladder can cause an infec-tion, so sitting in a diaper full of watery diarrhea or wiping "back to front" in little girls are ways to introduce bacteria into the urine.

While viral illnesses still account for the vast (vast!) majority of fevers in kids, UTIs are relatively common in young babies and children with fever. Some children with a more serious infection of the bladder and kidneys may have fever and vomiting. It isn't only an infection of the urine that can cause pain when going to the potty. Being constipated can put pressure on the bladder and cause either frequency (going very often), or pain when urinating. Constipation can even cause a true UTI, because urine doesn't completely drain from the compressed bladder and sits around, like stagnant water, allowing bacteria to grow. Being dehydrated can cause the urine to become very concentrated, which might be responsible for burning in some kids.

## She Refuses to Go

Urinating during the acute phase of a bladder infection can bring tears to a grown-up's eyes. Encourage plenty of fluids to dilute the urine and increase the volume. Appropriate doses of pain medication are important. In severe cases and for older kids, your doctor can prescribe a medication to numb the bladder. She may feel better sitting in a warm tub to pee, since the warm water will relax her and take some of the pain and pressure away.

If you are worried that your little one may have a UTI, then she is certainly going to need to see her doctor. Waiting until morning is most likely fine unless she is acting very ill, with vomiting, high fevers, or looking pretty sick. Your pediatrician can help you decide if a urine test can wait until morning or not. If the doctor determines that your child does, in fact, have a urinary tract infection, she will need to be treated with antibiotics. Kids who fail to respond to antibiotics by mouth or who are too sick or vomiting too frequently to take oral medication may require a hospital stay for IV treatment, but this is pretty rare. Once treated, most physicians recommend that certain tests be performed to ensure there is no reason for the UTI, especially in infants and boys. An ultrasound of the kidneys will ensure that the anatomy is normal,

## THE WORKUP

If your kid is diagnosed with a bladder or kidney infection, most physicians will recommend further evaluation to make sure the anatomy is normal and there is no physical reason for the infection. Repeated infections may go undetected and lead to significant and possibly permanent kidney damage. A renal ultrasound is a sonogram of the kidneys that is painless and easy. The ultrasound gives great information about the size, location, and number of kidneys but isn't good for evaluating urine flow or small anatomical abnormalities. A voiding cystourethrogram, or VCUG, is another test where special dye is inserted into the bladder via a catheter and then X-rays are taken to make sure the dye doesn't flow toward the kidneys, which is called urinary reflux. Both tests are important for determining whether a child is at risk for future infections or kidney problems and whether treatment is necessary.

while a special X-ray looking at dye put into the bladder evaluates the direction of urine flow and possible blockages. These tests will be arranged by your doctor as she feels necessary and are usually performed after the acute infection has been treated.

Urine testing should be done only on a clean urine sample. If your kiddo is not yet potty trained, this can be tricky. Sometimes a small baggie is placed over the wee one's privates in order to collect some pee. While this is the gentlest way to obtain urine, there is a high chance of contaminating the specimen with bacteria from the skin or anus. Therefore, it is generally considered standard of care that we obtain urine via a catheter whenever infection is a concern. While this sounds traumatic, it is vital that your physician be able to determine whether bacteria growing in the baby's urine came from the bladder or not.

## HOLDING THE BAG

Are you willing to commit your child to possibly years of antibiotics and invasive follow-up testing based on a falsely positive urine sample? Absolutely not. A urine specimen that is being examined for infection should be collected in a sterile manner. A sample obtained from a bag is useful only if it doesn't have any bacteria in it and is called negative by the lab.

The procedure is quite simple. After wiping the area clean, a very small, very soft, very flexible tube is inserted into the urethra and removed as soon as some urine is collected. The whole procedure takes just a few seconds. An alternative method is to insert a small needle directly into the bladder from the low abdomen. While this looks even more traumatic,

## YOU HAVE TO GO AGAIN?!

Some kids will develop a condition called frequency urgency syndrome of childhood. This delightful condition occurs when a previously well kid suddenly needs to urinate all the time, as often as every ten minutes. While this is extremely annoying, especially if you are staring at an upcoming family road trip, the condition is harmless and goes away over time. However, a doctor should see any child who develops a sudden increase in the frequency of urination to make sure there is no infection or other physical condition such as diabetes, which can present with increased thirst and urination. Once your pediatrician has cleared your kid of any medical causes of the urgent need to pee and you've addressed any other possible contributing factors such as constipation, there is nothing for you to do but wait. And teach your son to pee in a water bottle if you are still planning to take that cross-country drive.

it is actually a very safe and reliable method of obtaining a urine specimen. Depending on local practice, your physician may be more comfortable collecting urine in this fashion. I recommend you defer to your pediatrician on this issue.

## The Twig

### With or Without Foreskin

Circumcisions: Never mind the arguments for and against circumcision. If you have decided to leave Johnny's manlihood as it came, fine. We'll get to the care of the uncircumcised penis later. If, however, you've elected to have him circumcised, it was probably done when he was a newborn. There are some reasons why a circumcision is delayed until an infant is a bit older. Some babies are just a little too, um, petite at birth for the procedure, and we give those little critters a couple of months to, um, grow. Other babies are too ill in the newborn period and we don't want to add any additional stress. Sometimes parents are undecided. Or for whatever reason, the circumcision didn't happen at the hospital. So what should you know about having an older baby circumcised? After the newborn period, some pediatricians will perform the procedure in the office up until a certain age, usually a couple of months, when the baby is too big for the standard restraint device. Others will refer you to a urologist, or a doctor specializing in the male plumbing. Once a baby becomes a bit too big for the standard circumcision restraint equipment, the procedure is best done in the operating room, under general anesthesia.

Of note, sometimes a circumcision in the newborn period is started and an abnormality of the penis is discovered. This is most commonly an abnormal placement of the urethra,

## HURTING THE ONES YOU LOVE

If your bouncing baby boy is going to have his foreskin removed, no matter what his age, ask the doctor about pain control. Even brand-new babies should be offered local anesthesia in either a cream or injection. Sucking on a sugary pacifier during the procedure has also been shown to lessen the pain associated with medical procedures. Older babies should have oral pain medicine, such as acetaminophen, as well as anesthetic, whether local or general. Babies *do* feel pain. Don't believe otherwise.

or urine tube. In this case, the procedure is stopped immediately, no matter what may have already been cut. This is because we want to preserve as much foreskin as possible, so that the surgeon who performs the corrective surgery will have some extra skin to work with if needed.

## THAT'S ACTUALLY DISGUSTING

What many physicians forget to warn new parents about is that healing wounds can look a little gross. Remember that when a wound heals in a warm, moist environment (as on a penis), all those fabulous healing factors that come streaming in to promote rapid recovery take on a white, thick, junky look. This is normal and does not need to be removed.

Another word on baby penises when all is said and done: The circumcised penis needs to be gently yet thoroughly cleaned at every diaper change with the remaining foreskin gently retracted to allow visualization and cleansing of the entire glans. Otherwise, one of two things may happen. One is that the development of smegma can occur (yes, this is a real word; your buddies in junior high did not make it up), which is a collection of dead skin cells that build up in the space between the foreskin and the glans. The other possibility is the development of adhesions, or scar tissue, between the remaining foreskin and glans, making retraction of the foreskin impossible. Occasionally this is severe enough that the penis looks uncircumcised or, in the case of an exceptionally chubby young boy, may result in the near or complete disappearance of the penis into that little fat pad sitting right atop his little hoohah. This condition can be remedied, but in severe cases may require surgical correction. Or you can simply be a bit more vigilant at diaper time.

The uncircumcised foreskin should never be forcibly retracted during cleansing of the penis. On average, the foreskin becomes completely retractable by the age of four years, although some cannot completely retract theirs until puberty. Forceful retraction of a resistant foreskin will only cause pain, trauma, and possibly scar tissue, making the situation even worse.

If you notice foul-smelling drainage or redness spreading up the abdominal wall following a circumcision, quickly alert your physician. In addition, an uncircumcised male may develop a condition where the foreskin pulls back and gets "stuck" behind the glans, looking like a little foreskin balloon hat. This is a medical emergency and warrants immediate attention.

## Where Did It Go?

If you wake up one day and his penis seems to have disappeared, don't freak out. Little baby boys are often blessed with healthy rolls of fat, particularly in their suprapubic region, or the part over the bone that sits above the genitals. If this fat pad becomes big enough, it may appear to suck up the little penis. As long as you can free the penis from the surrounding skin and he can urinate normally, this isn't a problem and his boyhood will pop back out when he slims down.

### It's All Red

Most cases of a "red" penis are caused by local irritation of the glans, or tip of the penis. This is usually a result of either over- or undercleaning, vigorous manipulation, or possibly a bacterial infection. If your young chap wakes up to a sore, red penis, give him a gentle soak in the tub and see if a little tender care doesn't help. Your pediatrician may decide to prescribe an antibiotic by mouth or cream if the condition doesn't appear to be improving.

Rarely the foreskin of an uncircumcised penis can become trapped behind the glans, making the penis appear suddenly circumcised. The trapped foreskin can be quite red and tender. This condition is called paraphimosis and is considered an emergency, since the trapped foreskin may lose its blood supply if not returned to its natural position.

Whether the foreskin appears trapped or the penis simply appears red, don't take chances with his one and only. If the foreskin is easily movable (or he doesn't have one) and the redness is confined to just the tip of the penis, wait a day or so and try some gentle cleaning and protection. However, a trapped foreskin, redness extending up the shaft of the penis or onto the belly, or an inability to urinate should prompt a quick call to your pediatrician.

## The Berries

### Where Are They?

Remember that a full-term newborn boy will have a scrotum that is more adultlike in appearance. The testicles will hang low and the skin will be quite loose. However, as Mom's hormones clear from his body, the skin will tighten up and the scrotum will generally shrink in size and lie closer to the body.

Of common concern to many parents is: Where's the testicle? There are a couple of conditions that may make it more difficult to find both testicles in an infant. One is the retractile testicle. This is a testicle that prefers to sit up in the canal leading back into the body. When a little boy fetus is developing, the testicles sit up inside the belly and then descend into the scrotum through a little tunnel. Normally this small canal seals up and keeps the belly cavity and the scrotum from sharing occupants such as bowel or fluid. A retractile testicle is not actually going back into the belly, but just sitting in the remnant of that tunnel. If your doctor starts at the top of the scrotum and pushes down, the testicle will pop into the lower scrotum and can be found easily. Placing the baby in warm water will also encourage a shy testicle to descend, which is the preferred "at home" method to ensure there are really two of them.

A testicle that is never in the scrotum and cannot be found by either of the above methods is referred to as an undescended testicle. Here the testicle just failed to make the trip down south and is still sitting up in the belly. This is a surgically corrected procedure and does require attention. While not an emergency, most surgeons will retrieve the testicle and place it in the scrotum before one year of age. In case you are wondering, the testicle would work fine in either place. But there may be a slightly higher risk of testicular cancer for an undescended testicle. The risk does not change by placing it back in the scrotum, but it does give a young man the ability to "self-examine" and promote early evaluation of any abnormal lumps or firmness to the testicle.

## The Size

How about a scrotum that seems more full, or uneven? It is quite common to have a collection of fluid, called a hydrocele, filling one or both sides of the scrotum. This fluid will eventually dry up and shouldn't cause a problem, although your pediatrician will want to take a look. More rarely the little canal through which the testicles descended will fail to close completely. This allows fluid to travel between the scrotum and the belly. So, if the swelling seems to be intermittent, please let your pediatrician know. If this opening in the canal is large enough, bowel loops can actually slip through and sit in the scrotum. This is what is commonly referred to as a hernia. This will eventually need surgical correction. As

### EMERGENCY!

If the swelling in the scrotum ever seems very hard or red, if the baby seems to be in pain or has repeated vomiting, he needs to be evaluated by a medical professional immediately. Rarely, the loops of bowel become so tightly packed in that they can't slip back out. This cuts off the bowel's blood supply and becomes what we refer to as an incarcerated hernia. This condition requires immediate attention before the trapped piece of bowel begins to die from a lack of oxygen and has to be removed.

long as the swelling can be gently compressed back up into the belly by your doctor, surgery can wait until the baby is a bit bigger and better able to handle anesthesia and a surgical procedure.

## EMERGENCY!

Any kid with acute pain or tenderness of a testicle needs to be seen by his doctor urgently. While rare in really little kids, it is still possible for a condition called testicular torsion to occur, which is when the testicle twists around, cutting off its own blood supply. If the testicle isn't untwisted and fixed back into place in the scrotum, it could die within as little as several hours. Call your doctor.

### Penile and Scrotal Trauma

There is actually an entire chapter in my emergency procedures textbook regarding the removal of a penis from a zipper. I suppose it actually applies to any skin caught up in said mechanism, but speaking from experience, the penis is the most likely victim. So you can see, injuries to the penis and scrotum are not that rare. Fortunately, only a few require emergency treatment.

Blunt trauma refers to injury that comes from a forceful blow, such as being kicked in the groin. A significant blow to the scrotum can, rarely, lead to impressive bleeding and swelling. If the scrotum appears very bruised or swollen, you should call your pediatrician because it may be necessary to evaluate the testicles using an ultrasound. However, for most blunt blows to the privates, as long as you can feel each testicle and they seem normal and your kid is able to urinate, there is nothing to do.

Crush injuries occur when a forceful blow results in injury to the skin and underlying structures. Short little kids can sustain such an injury from a falling toilet seat or lid. Talk about a blow to your toilet training efforts. Literally. Fortunately most of these injuries are pretty minor, and as long as there is only a small scratch and no large cut and your child can still urinate, nothing more than perhaps a bit of antibiotic ointment is necessary.

For all injuries to the genitals, as long as bleeding is controlled and the kid can tinkle, there is rarely a need for emergency evaluation. Call your pediatrician if you aren't sure. If your child is refusing to pee because of pain, plop him in a warm tub and encourage him to urinate in the water once he's relaxed. And as with any injury, report any signs of infection, such as increasing pain, redness, or swelling, to your doctor.

### ZIPPER INJURIES

If your child makes the unfortunate mistake of trying to get dressed and out the door too quickly, you may find yourself facing a bit of a dilemma. Try unzipping the zipper once. If that doesn't work, you can try cutting the zipper out of the clothing and manually pulling the teeth apart from the other side. If your kid will let you near his genitals with a wire cutter, find the metal bar at the top of the slider (handle) that runs across to both sides of the slider and snip it. This will make the slider fall off and will release the zipper entirely. Alternatively, slice right across the teeth of the zipper above or below the caught skin and pull the teeth apart. If you can't free the skin despite your best efforts, call your doctor. Probably now, since your kid won't be sleeping with his skin stuck in the zipper.

## It's a Girl

### A Bump or a Lump

Let's say you find a firm little lump in the skin folds next to the vagina. This needs to be brought to the attention of your physician but is not emergent. Rarely, an ovary migrates south along the canal intended for a testicle. This also needs surgical correction and an evaluation by a physician as this condition may (but probably not!) indicate some additional abnormalities.

A pretty rare but weird thing in a girl's privates that may prompt parents to panic is a blockage of the vagina. In cases where there is skin covering the outlet of the vagina, fluid and material may build up behind the blockage, eventually causing a bulging lump to appear. As long as the baby can urinate and appears otherwise well, this is not an emergency, but you should let your doctor know (during regular business hours).

### Where Did Her Vagina Go?

What if the area around the vagina looks "stuck together"? The folds of skin outside the vagina are called the labia. Until puberty hits, the skin there is thicker and doesn't have as much moisture. So, sometimes, the skin of the vulva can actually stick to the vulva on the other side, effectively sealing up the vagina. This is called a labial adhesion. Most babies with labial adhesions have no symptoms and the condition fixes itself at puberty, when the female hormone, estrogen, makes the skin thinner and more lubricated. However, some children will have trouble urinating. And a lot of parents just don't like it. If your doctor decides to treat the adhesions, daily application of a cream containing estrogen will generally fix the problem within a couple of weeks.

## PAIN DOWN THERE

No matter the cause—be it irritation, infection, or trauma—of pain in the privates, little kids will hold their pee until their eyes turn yellow. All kids are more relaxed in a warm tub of water and this might be the only place you can get her to pee for a few days until things are better.

## Vaginal Bleeding

After the newborn period, any bleeding from the vagina should be considered abnormal and evaluated by your doctor during regular office hours unless the bleeding is extremely heavy (soaking underwear). However, what appears to be bleeding from the vagina might actually be something entirely different. One cause of small amounts of blood is called urethral prolapse. This is when the first little bit of the tube that leads to the bladder (the urethra) flips inside out. The inside lining of the urethra is very fragile and easily irritated, so the only symptom may be spotting of blood in the underwear. A little girl may also complain of pain, especially when urinating. A prolapsed urethra will look like a little bright red donut sitting below the clitoris and above the entrance to the vagina. This is not an emergency and would eventually correct itself. However, because it can be painful and cause bleeding and irritation, an estrogen-containing cream can be prescribed, which will encourage the inside-out skin to return to its normal location. In the meantime, let her soak in a warm tub a couple of times a day to gently clean the area, avoiding soaps or bubble baths. If the pain is making it diffi-cult to urinate, let her pee in the tub.

## Discharge

A certain amount of discharge from the vagina can be normal even in prepubescent kids. A thin, watery discharge is called leukorrhea and is completely normal. Any discharge that is colored or accompanied by surrounding redness or itch-ing needs to be evaluated by your pediatrician, although it is very unlikely to be an emergency. Many little girls will develop painful or itchy irritation due to either poor hygiene or contact with irritating substances, such as bubble baths. When the skin of the vagina and surrounding area is irritated but there is no infection present, we call that nonspecific vul-vovaginitis. Make sure she is using clean cotton undies (even if that means you have to buy five pairs of the pink Minnie Mouse ones) and avoid snug tights or synthetic materials that may trap moisture and not allow the skin to breathe. Also avoid the use of soap, bubble baths, or lotions. If your tot is very uncomfortable, a warm soak in the tub followed by a quick drying with a cool-set hair dryer and a smearing of diaper cream will make her feel better and let you get some sleep.

## Is That a Lego?!

Little girls like to explore the world just as much as little boys. Trouble is, they have one extra hole in which to stick something that doesn't belong. Toilet tissue is the most com-monly found foreign body of the vagina, although I one time had to fish out some pennies. No matter what part of the body a foreign substance sits in, the immune system will eventually recognize it as "not self" and attempt to get rid of it. A foul smell or greenish-colored discharge may be the only sign of a foreign body in a little girl's vagina. If you do see something there that doesn't belong, it is likely going to require some expert maneuvering to retrieve it without hurting the poor kid, so give your doctor a call.

## Trauma

Seems like nearly every female I know has, at one time or another in her childhood, sustained an injury to her privates. A "saddle injury" refers to a cut, scrape, or bruise that can occur when a little girl inadvertently falls or is hit with something (such as a bike bar!) in the genitals. These injuries are extremely common and almost never require emergency treatment, although occasionally a little girl will hurt herself badly enough to require evaluation and treatment. However, the vast majority of little girls will heal up just fine without any intervention whatsoever. If your little gymnast falls on the balance beam, a little bleeding in the underwear is okay. If the bleeding doesn't stop shortly, or is very heavy or full of clots, she is going to need to see someone. Put a maxi-pad or towel between her legs and give your pediatrician a call. If the bleeding is easily controlled, just be certain that she can urinate. Because the injury is painful, she may refuse to use the toilet. In that case, try having her sit in a warm tub and pee in the water. If your best cajoling and offer of bribes don't get you anywhere, give your doc a call, but chances are that everything is just fine.

# the body, arms, and legs

This chapter is about everything from the neck all the way to the little piggies. Except the skin and organs. So I guess it's about fat, muscles, bones, tendons, ligaments, and everything else that makes up both the framework over which his sweet baby skin hangs and the cage that holds all of his important parts.

## The Neck

### A Bump

The number one worry parents have about their child's neck is when they find a lump or a bump. The human body is very intelligent in design and has little infection battle stations built in at various points in the body. The lymph nodes are some of the battle stations and can be found in chains along the scalp and neck, under the armpits, and along the groin. When an infection or some other form of irritation occurs, the white blood cells in our body (the cells that fight infection) travel to the site of the problem and then report back to the nearest lymph node for a debriefing and recruitment of other infection fighters. In the neck, these lymph nodes feel like rubbery little balls that move under your fingers. They may be about the size of a pea and grow as big as a large cherry tomato when fighting infection. Sometimes these nodes can be tender, especially when inflamed.

Occasionally one of the lymph nodes itself will get infected and will become much larger, maybe the size of an egg. The skin may also become very red. These infected nodes generally need antibiotics and you should see your pediatrician tomorrow.

If your child has a swelling in his neck that you think is a lymph node, but doesn't move, is very hard, or doesn't seem to be tender, call your pediatrician. This is an unusual occurrence and one that we want to know about.

Most important, if there is swelling of the side of the neck *and* your baby refuses to turn her head, especially if there is fever, call your doctor. An irritable baby with a fever and refusal to turn her head may have developed a pus pocket, or abscess, in the tissues of the neck. These infections require IV antibiotics and sometimes must be drained. These abscesses might be so deep into the neck that there is no visible swelling or redness. Drooling or refusing to drink might occur because her throat is sore. So, any fever coupled with a refusal to turn her head is cause for worry until proven otherwise. A call to your doctor at midnight would be appropriate in this case.

## SHE WON'T TURN HER HEAD

A kid who refuses to turn her head may have only a muscle spasm and it would be okay to try an age-appropriate dose of pain medicine and some warm, moist heat or a little massage. *But* if there are any other symptoms, such as drooling or refusing liquids, *or* if there is a fever of any kind, call your doctor immediately.

Finally, there are plenty of other little lumps and bumps that may appear along the sides or front of the neck. These may be little remnants of the various ridges and holes and whatnot that appear during early fetal development. Depending on where it is, how big it is, and whether it becomes infected, your doctor will know whether it is something that needs to be removed or ignored. Just mention it at the next appointment.

## He Can't Turn His Head

Just like we can get a crick in our neck, so can babies. Some babies are born with a tight muscle in their neck, called torticollis, while others may develop it later. Torticollis means an abnormal positioning of the head, usually turned and slightly tilted to one side. Generally, gentle stretching, warm compresses, and time are all that is needed, but your doctor should see your baby to make sure this is nothing more than a muscle spasm. Older babies and young children can develop torticollis after a mild injury. If there is *no* pain along the bones in the center of the neck, she can move her fingers and toes, and seems to have normal strength all over, this is usually just a spasm of the muscle and will also respond to pain medicine (such as ibuprofen), warm compresses, and gentle massage. If you in any way think that there is more going on than a simple muscle spasm, if she has any pain over the bones of the neck, or if she is limping, not using one arm or leg, or seems weak, call your doctor immediately.

Any refusal to move her head every which way combined with a fever means you are making a phone call. This is a situation that needs more urgent evaluation and you shouldn't hesitate to call your pediatrician right now. An infection of the

fluid protecting the brain and spinal column is called meningitis and can cause pain with movement of the neck along
with other signs of infection, such as fever and vomiting. Little
babies may just cry or be extremely irritable when picked up
or moved, while older babies and kids may turn into stiff
boards, refusing to bend any part of the neck or back. Any
fever accompanied by severe irritability, confusion, or a refusal
to move (that isn't remedied with a dose of a pain- and fever-
relieving medication) requires an urgent call to your doctor.

## Neck Injuries

Everyone knows that the neck contains the most important part of our spinal column, where all the nerves live that
control how we move and feel. An injury to the spinal
column up in the neck may affect our ability to move our
whole body, or even to breathe. Scary, eh? The good news is
that kids rarely injure the bones or nerves of the neck. That
said, in small children the head is so big in proportion to the
rest of the body, that certain high-speed movements may
cause high neck, or cervical, spine injuries. Examples would
include a small baby being grabbed by the skull during a dog
attack and flung around like a rag doll. Sitting in a front-
facing car seat before his neck muscles are strong enough to
control his head during a car accident (at least one year of
age), or being hit by an airbag while sitting in the front seat,
are other ways in which small kids can injure their necks.
That's why your kid sits in the back until he is the one
buying the car.

For all other kids, short of falling straight onto his head
from up in a tree or diving into shallow water, cervical spine
injuries are pretty rare. If your kid falls down and bounces

right back up, she's probably fine. No baby or toddler is going to lie motionless on the ground unless truly injured. If she jumps up and runs to you, no worries. For a slightly older kiddo who has fallen and is now complaining of neck pain, make sure that his arms and legs are moving and he looks otherwise normal. If he willingly moves his neck in all directions (not *you* forcing his head to turn!), and has no pain along the bones in the middle, try a dose of ibuprofen. If you are in doubt at all, call your pediatrician. Any child who has injured his neck and complains, either at the time or later, of tingling or numbness in the arms or legs, has weakness, is potty trained but suddenly having accidents, or exhibits anything else out of the ordinary, call your doctor right away.

## 911!

If your child has fallen, or otherwise may have injured his neck, and is not moving or unconscious, do *not* move him unless he is in imminent danger of further injury. Call 911 immediately. If he is crying and awake but not getting up on his own, leave him be and call 911. You might want to try to stabilize the neck in the *position in which you found it*, say with your hands or a couple of sweaters or towels placed next to his head and neck, to keep his head from rolling or his neck from moving. It is very important never to move the neck of someone who may have sustained an injury to the spinal cord because the movement might cause a partial injury to become complete or permanent.

If your kid has taken a blow to the front of the neck, such as from an errant game of "catch," and is able to talk normally and isn't having trouble breathing (aside from the initial crying fit), he is probably okay. It would be rare that being hit across the neck could cause enough injury and bruising to begin to press in on the airway.

> ⊖ | | !
>
> Any rapid swelling, change in voice, or difficulty breathing after a neck injury demands a call to 911.

## The Arms and Legs

### She Won't Move Her Arm

If your baby sustained an injury to the nerves of the arm during delivery (see "The Waiter's Tip," on page 15), you've probably already noticed this. If, however, she is suddenly refusing to move one hand or arm, an injury is the most likely cause. In the absence of an obvious source of pain, the most common of these injuries is a nursemaid elbow.

Babies have nice loosey-goosey joints, which give them great flexibility but also means that things don't always stick the way they are supposed to. In babies and small children, a pull on the arm can cause the bones of the elbow to pop up and over the ligament holding the elbow together. We call it a nursemaid elbow because it classically occurs when someone (the nursemaid) pulls a child by the hand to get him to come along. But I've seen babies do it to themselves just rolling across the floor. Toddlers fighting getting into their jammies at bedtime can get one. And how I cringe at the playground when I see someone swinging a toddler around by his hands. Sometimes there is no good explanation for a nursemaid elbow (or radial subluxation). All of a sudden, a baby or small child will refuse to use one arm, generally holding it sort of flexed, or bent, at the elbow. He'll cry when you try to move his arm, and if he is old enough to tell you where it hurts, he will point to his wrist.

I *love* this diagnosis, because I know exactly what is wrong and I can fix it immediately, which is a rarity in my line of work. To fix a nursemaid elbow, we do this fancy little maneuver that is a trade secret. Actually, I won't tell you how because sometimes it is difficult to know whether a nursemaid elbow is actually a broken bone and manipulating the arm could cause more damage. So, call your pediatrician and tell her that you suspect your child has a nursemaid elbow. She might walk you through the way to fix it if there is no swelling, tenderness, or bruising, but she'll probably send you my way if her office has already closed for the day.

## THE MAGIC X-RAY

Nursemaid elbows are extremely common and are easily fixed by manipulating the ligament back over the bone. It is quite a common occurrence for a kid who is sent immediately to radiology to return from his X-rays "all better," because the radiology technician inadvertently corrected the problem while positioning the arm for the pictures. So, it might be better to see the doctor *first* and not just run straight to X-rays if your kid might have a nursemaid elbow. Save him a little radiation.

### Is It Broken?

Because a child's bones are still forming, they are quite soft as compared to those of an adult. And they are pretty weak compared to the tissues that connect them. Therefore, while adults are more likely to injure the ligaments and tendons that hold our muscles and bones together, children are more likely to break a bone. What's more, kids have very soft areas in key positions on the bones, called growth plates, which allow for their bodies to grow and change with time. Damage to the growth center could mean that growth is stunted or abnormal.

Because an injury in a child is more likely to be a broken bone than a simple sprain, and because we have to be very careful with the delicate growth plates, any injury that causes pain over the bone should be considered a fracture until proven otherwise. In fact, because the growth plates don't show up well on X-ray, pain over a growth plate should be considered a fracture even with a normal radiograph.

Refusing to use an arm or leg, swelling of an area over a bone, or crying when picked up or moved are all clues that a bone may have been broken. Call your pediatrician if you are worried about any of these symptoms. In other words, if your child has fallen and injured himself and continues to complain of pain, limps, or has swelling or bruising over a bone, call your doctor. Clearly not all of these kids need to be seen in the ER, but depending on the type of injury, the age of the child, and where the pain is, an X-ray and possibly a referral to a bone doctor, or orthopedist, may be warranted.

If your child does just seem to have sprained or strained one of his tentacles, ibuprofen will help with both the pain and swelling. An ice pack wrapped in a towel (never directly in contact with the skin!) for twenty minutes or so as tolerated is also fine. Any cold, blue, or numb fingers or toes should be reported to your pediatrician immediately.

## Oh Yeah, It's Broken

If a broken bone, or fracture (these are the same thing!), is pretty obvious, you'll want to get your child to the ER in a

## Is It Broken or Sprained?

Young children are more likely to break a bone than have a simple sprain. "Point tenderness" is how we describe the pain associated with a fracture and it means pain over one specific spot (i.e., the broken part). Significant pain in a joint or over a bone warrants a call to your doctor. Pain over the "whole arm" that doesn't hurt in any one place more than anywhere else is most likely just bruised. Or, as I teach the medical students, if "everything" hurts, "nothing" is broken.

timely fashion. If it is impossible to move him without causing serious pain, go ahead and call an ambulance. If there is bleeding or a cut on the injured limb, we are going to assume that the bone poked through the skin at the time of the injury, which is called an open fracture. Open fractures are very high-risk injuries because they easily become infected. Unfortunately, the cuts in the skin are most commonly extremely subtle, as just a sharp tip of a bone pushes into the skin before sliding back down into its final resting place. If you see any

## Stabilizing the Injury

Splinting an injury before moving a child is generally a good idea. *Splinting* means bracing the injured part to prevent further movement. A good splint will significantly reduce a child's pain and make transport to the ER a whole lot easier. Rolled-up newspaper and masking tape make a pretty good splint. So do magazines, straight rulers, and cardboard. Be sure to pad the injured area pretty well, maybe with a kitchen towel. And try not to apply tape directly to his skin, because when they pull it off, he'll be really mad.

bleeding or cuts, gently cover the wound with a clean cloth and be sure to tell the ER staff about it when you arrive.

What is most important if you are going to the ER because you think your child has broken a bone is *not* to give him anything to eat or drink until the ER staff has said it is okay. If the bones are not in perfect or near-perfect position, they may have to be moved, or set, before being put in a cast or splint. Most children who require manipulation of their bones will receive medicine to make them sleepy and provide pain control. These medicines are best given on an empty stomach, as vomiting is not only unpleasant, but may go into the lungs of a sleepy, not totally "with it," kid. In some hospitals, the staff will actually wait until a child has been four, six, or even eight hours without food or drink before administering the necessary medications. This is a safety issue and we take it very seriously. So he should have *nothing*. No water. No ice. No candy. No lollipop. No chewing gum. Nothing means nothing. I don't care if he is hungry. You can survive hunger. But food in your lungs can be very, very serious. The ER staff will be more than happy to let you know when it is safe for your child to eat or drink. Heck, they'll probably be so grateful that they'll round up some crackers and pudding for you.

## Limp

By about nine months, most babies are able to pull to a stand and will begin "cruising" around furniture shortly thereafter. By one year of age, many babies are able to take a few tottering steps on their own, although it isn't outside the range of normal if yours hasn't gotten there yet! By eighteen months, most kids are tearing around the house, mobile enough to destroy your belongings, too young to understand their value. Delightful combination.

What to do if your baby suddenly seems to avoid using one leg or is refusing to walk when she could just yesterday? There are many causes of a limp in little ones. An injury is the likeliest culprit. Without any history of injury or any obvious swelling, something called a toddler's fracture, which is a fracture (or break in the bone) of the tibia, or the main shinbone, is relatively common. A toddler's fracture can occur without significant force and is usually the result of an active little kid getting a touch carried away with himself. The break in the bone can be difficult to find, even on X-ray, so sometimes we will put a suspected fracture in a cast and send him to see an orthopedist, even when the films are normal. As for other broken bones, those are usually a little more obvious, with pain, swelling, and bruising at the site of the injury.

A rock in his shoe could be another reason for limping. Pain from either a foreign body, such as a splinter, or another injury, such as a blister on the foot, may also be to blame. If your child is limping or refusing to walk, take off her shoes. Look at the bottoms of her feet and between her toes. If you see an area of irritation, redness, or swelling, you may have solved the case. Try changing shoes or bandaging the wound. If you suspect that a small sliver of wood, glass, or other for-

## SAND IN MY SHOE

When I was about three, I kept complaining of sand in my shoe and refusing to walk. It took my mother a good couple of times removing my footwear and inspecting my foot before she realized that my leg had fallen asleep. It's just a thought.

eign material is to blame, and you can't easily (easily!) find or remove the object, call your pediatrician. We would rather try to take a foreign object out of the skin *before* you have dug around and turned it into a bloody mess.

Infections in a joint may cause redness and swelling of the affected joint or just pain with movement. Most kids with an infected joint will have a fever. All suspected joint infections are considered emergencies, as are infections of the bones. So, if your baby appears ill, or has a fever or vomiting in addition to what appears to be a painful joint or limp, call your doctor immediately.

> ## WARNING!
>
> A child with a limp *and* a fever, or a kid with redness or swelling of a joint, needs to be seen by a doctor. An infection of the bone or fluid in the joint can cause serious, possibly permanent damage, and requires early and aggressive management. Call your pediatrician now.

But if she is happy as a clam and not sick at all, other than refusing to walk, you can relax a bit. Some babies will develop a condition called toxic synovitis, or a cold in the hip. This occurs usually after a viral infection and is thought to be an inflammation of the hip joint by the immune system. Think of it as if all the cells fighting the cold got to go on vacation down in the hip after their work was done. Kids with toxic synovitis are generally pretty well and happy, don't have fever, and just refuse to walk. A dose of an anti-inflammatory medication, such as ibuprofen, will often provide tremendous relief. The condition goes away by itself in about a week. However, your pediatrician will definitely want to know if you think your kid has toxic synovitis, because we need to be absolutely certain that he does not actually have a potentially serious joint infection instead.

## Swollen Joints

As mentioned above under "Limp," on page 169, joints such as the hips, knees, or elbows may become infected in babies and children. If your child refuses to move a joint, especially if there is redness and swelling, or if she appears otherwise unwell, with fever or perhaps vomiting, she should be seen promptly by a doctor. Call your pediatrician.

## Fingers and Toes

Curious little fingers go everywhere. As a result, injuries or infections of the nails and surrounding skin are pretty common in little kids. Be it a finger or a toe, the rules are pretty much the same. An infection of the area around the nail is called a paronychia and may cause redness, swelling, and pain. Sometimes the infection will have matured enough to produce a pocket of pus. Paronychia are often the result of ingrown toenails or from biting or picking at the cuticle of the fingernail. To prevent such a painful infection, keep toenails cut straight across, not down on the sides where they can grow into the tender flesh around your kiddo's toes. Cuticles on the hands can generally be left alone, but clip any ragged or torn bits with a nail clipper and try to keep your kid from chewing on them. If an infection does occur, you can try to have her soak the affected digit in warm water. If she won't go for that, warm compresses, such as a warm, wet washcloth, might help any infection to drain. At the very least, you can pop her whole self into the tub for a while. If the finger or toe doesn't start to look better within a day or two, you're probably going to have to see your doctor. Sometimes a piece of the nail needs removing to allow the infection to drain properly.

Any door, be it in the house or on your car, can catch an unsuspecting finger. Heavy objects seem to seek out toes when dropped. Injuries to fingers and toes can be scary, especially if part of the skin or bone has been crushed. An injury to the nail can cause bleeding under the nail, which is called a subungual hematoma. These can be very painful, because the blood collecting under the nail causes a lot of pressure on the tip of the finger or toe. A hematoma under the nail will look dark and be pretty obvious. If the darkened area is big enough, your doctor might choose to drain the blood by creating a very small hole in the nail. This actually doesn't hurt and gives immediate relief of the terrible throbbing pain. The nail may be a little abnormal looking until the injured part has grown back out, but with time should be fine.

Occasionally an injury of the nail will cause a cut in the skin underneath, which often requires emergency care. Sometimes we have to remove the nail to repair the cut. Very often the new nail will grow in normally, but sometimes the damage to the nail plate is more substantial and a new nail won't grow, or will grow abnormally.

An injury that involves the skin, and possibly bone, of the fingertip is not uncommon in little kids. Any of these injuries, except for the most minor of bruises, is going to require a phone call to your doctor and probably a trip to the ER. Rest assured that even the most horrible-looking injuries to the fingertips often heal surprisingly well in children. But remember to be vigilant about checking the whereabouts of all fingers and toes before closing car and house doors.

## The Torso

### Bumps

Remember back to "The Neck," on pages 158–59, when we talked about the lymph nodes? We all have infection-fighting centers that run in chains in various places of the body. These centers are where the cells that fight infection gather to discuss game strategy. Chains of lymph nodes are found all around the neck and scalp, but they also occur elsewhere, notably in the groin and armpits. As in the neck, they may become larger and increasingly tender if fighting a nearby infection or inflammation. Occasionally one of the lymph nodes itself will get infected, and the node will become much larger. The skin may also become very red.

Lymph nodes in the armpits can't generally be felt but might become big enough to see or feel if the node itself becomes infected or if there is an infection somewhere on the arm. If a lymph node in the armpit becomes very red and tender, or you notice a swelling that is continuing to grow, especially if it doesn't hurt, make an appointment to see your doctor tomorrow.

The groin is the area at the top of the legs, just over the hips. Babies are usually so fat that you can't find your way to the bottom of it, but as kids get a little bigger and a little leaner, you can often feel the lymph nodes along this line. Once again, there is nothing to worry about as long as there is no redness of the overlying skin, implying that a node has become infected. Also, we want to know about *any* lump that is growing with time, particularly if it is not tender, doesn't move, or feels very hard.

There is one last place where a lymph node may pop up and that is along the elbow, on the side closest to the body.

Any infection of the hand or forearm could cause these lymph nodes to become enlarged, but one particular infection that is associated with cat and kitten scratches may present in such a fashion. This infection does require antibiotics, so your doctor might want to check for it using a specific blood test.

## LUMPS AND BUMPS

A lymph node that is growing with time, very hard, and doesn't move under your fingertips needs to be brought to the attention of your doctor. Same for nodes that are very red, extremely swollen, and tender. Tenderness itself is pretty normal. Tender *and* red and swollen need an evaluation.

## Belly Buttons

Belly buttons. Whether an "outie" or an "innie," by now your baby has lost her umbilical cord (if not, call your doctor) and is proudly displaying her true belly button. But of course you still have questions. What is that funny little fleshy thing growing out from its center? Some babies will develop something called a pyogenic granuloma. This looks like a small stalk of abnormal skin protruding from the base of the umbilicus after the cord has fallen off and is occasionally prone to bleeding when irritated. It is also normal and will fall off with time. Your physician can also hasten its disappearance using a small amount of silver nitrate to chemically burn, or cauterize, it at the base. However, this isn't necessary and it will usually fall off on its own before swimsuit season.

Small umbilical hernias are quite common. The space in the muscles around the belly button in some kids is just a little larger and air and intestines can poke through. As a kid

## THE COIN

An old wives' tale involves taping a coin over the umbilical hernia to keep it flat and make it grow smaller. Because a kid will eventually "grow into" her hernia, the coin trick works only if you don't look under it for two or three years.

grows, the hole will stay the same size, meaning that she will eventually grow into her belly button and it won't look so big. It is extremely rare that an umbilical hernia needs to be corrected surgically. A very large hernia that persists after she starts school may need repair for cosmetic reasons. Even less common is to have a piece of bowel become stuck in the space and become strangulated. This is called an incarcerated hernia and would require immediate attention. An umbilical hernia that is soft and can be pushed back in easily is nothing to worry about. Extreme pain, redness, or hardness of the hernia should prompt a quick call to your doctor.

Rarely, a belly button might have an abnormal connection to the organs of the belly. Please let your doctor know if there is any persistent drainage of any type coming from the umbilicus. As long as there is no redness and the drainage isn't thick and green or yellow, like pus, this can probably wait until

## EMERGENCY!

The following are absolutely not normal: any foul-smelling or discolored drainage from a baby's umbilicus is cause for concern. In addition, any redness, warmth, or tenderness extending onto the belly should sound alarms. Call your doctor immediately.

morning. Any signs of infection, however, require a midnight phone call.

> ## Is That a Potato Plant?
>
> If your kid is a little older and has always had a completely normal belly button, but suddenly you think you see something abnormal in there, stick her in the tub. It's probably dirt.

## Backache

Unlike grown-ups, "backache" is a very uncommon complaint in toddlers and young children. If your kid is complaining of a backache today and yesterday she was having a great time in tumbling class, then it is okay to try a dose of pain medicine and wait and see. But if a child is complaining of back pain regularly, your pediatrician absolutely wants you to call him. Finally, remember that fever can give you aches and pains everywhere, including in your back. But if a kid is complaining of back pain and has a fever, especially if the pain is not entirely relieved with a reduction in the fever, you need to call your doctor. A child who is already potty trained and suddenly is having accidents also needs a good look-over. If in doubt, don't hesitate to let your doctor in on your worries.

> ## Emergency!
>
> If a child who is complaining of pain in his back also develops weakness of the legs, a limp, trouble running, or seems clumsier than usual, this is something that needs to be seen in an urgent fashion.

# the skin

Our skin is the largest, and some would say most important, organ of the body. It keeps us from leaking our fluids all over the couch. It is loaded with sensitive nerve endings and very helpfully lets us know when our pants are pinching or when someone is giving us a nice back scratch. But because there is so much of it, our skin, or dermis, is often the first place where infection or inflammation, either locally or within the whole body, will become evident. While an entire book couldn't cover every rash or spot that can appear on a kid, I will cover some of the more common rashes that pop up in the middle of the night and freak parents out.

## Rash

### When to Worry

Most rashes in babies and young children are pretty common and no cause for panic. The vast majority of rashes are of no consequence, and many are viral in nature. Remember, if your child otherwise looks well, is happy and playful, eating and drinking, and isn't bothered by the rash, life is good. In fact, there are only a few times when a rash is a sign of serious illness or needs emergency attention. A child who is acting very ill, even when his fever is brought down, needs to be seen urgently, as does a kid with a stiff neck, severe headache, or confusion or inappropriateness. Don't focus on the rash; focus on your kid.

## Diaper Rash

This is the biggie. Most diaper rashes can be divided into one of two categories: irritant or yeast. Irritant, or contact, diaper rashes are the result of urine and stool sitting in that nice warm, dark, superleakproof diaper. After a while, skin breakdown and irritation occur. Some babies are actually sensitive to materials in the diapers. The key to treating (or preventing!) most cases of diaper rash is simple: clean, dry, and protected. Frequent diaper changing and thorough cleansing are essential. The most expensive baby wipe on the market is not. A washcloth will do. But wash thoroughly. This means in between those little layers of baby fat and all around. (Remember for little girls, wipe front to back!) Then dry. If you have a very delicate, rash-prone baby, a hairdryer on cool will speed the process along. Then protect. Any good barrier cream, such as Desitin or A&D, will work. A good diaper cream should have a metal component, such as magnesium or

### KEEPING IT DRY

If your kid has a diaper rash of any kind and can run naked, that would be ideal. Letting the area dry out and have a break from the diapers and the poop and pee that fill them is a great idea. If, however, you want to go out in public or just got a new carpet, try drying the area with a hairdryer set on cool to make sure the skin is absolutely dry before applying your protective creams.

aluminum, as well as provide a good waterproof barrier between baby's skin and all that "output." In fact, I often recommend a good wiping with an antacid. Most liquid antacids have the same ingredients as diaper cream. I had one mother swear by cherry-flavored Maalox. The benefit is that it is probably already in your refrigerator and you can pour yourself a little swig at the same time.

The second type of common diaper rash is due to yeast. We all have yeast growing on our bodies that is normally kept in check by good bacteria. Sometimes, however, the yeast starts growing out of control and makes trouble. Taking antibiotics, for example, kills good and bad bacteria without discrimination, meaning yeast can grow unchecked. Yeast also loves a warm, dark, moist place. Like a diaper. A yeast rash differs from a contact rash by the presence of small "satellite" lesions. These are tiny red dots spreading out from the edge of the rash. Also, a yeasty rash will be worse in the folds of the skin, where it is warm, dark, and damp, as opposed to a contact-type rash, which is worse on the areas that are in contact with the offending material. As with all diaper rashes, the key is keeping everything clean and dry. Just go back and reread the previous paragraph. The biggest difference between an irritant rash and a rash caused by yeast is that an antifungal medication is needed. This can be a prescription medication or you can use an over-the-counter preparation such as clotrimazole. Check with your pediatrician as to those preparations that are safe to use on your sensitive and soft, albeit yeasty, baby's bottom.

Another type of diaper rash is actually an extension of seborrhea, or cradle cap. This rash will be very red and greasy in appearance. The clue to making this diagnosis is that the baby will also have a flaky rash of the scalp and the rash should also be present on the body, heading south to the diaper area. This will go away with time, or treating the cradle cap can speed the process along. Keep reading.

A rash that appears to be very red and is accompanied by little pimples or large blisters needs to be evaluated urgently. This may indicate a bacterial infection, which will require antibiotics and careful observation.

## Rashes of the Scalp

Cradle cap, also known as seborrhea, is a very common rash that first appears on the scalp, although it can progress all the way down south to the toes. For most babies, this is nothing more than a few flakes on the scalp, maybe a "greasy" red rash on the forehead and a few flakes in the eyebrows. Seborrhea can be treated or you can just leave it alone and it will go away with time. While some of my colleagues are fans of the latter strategy (why complicate things?), I am vain enough that I can understand not wanting a greasy, flaky, red infant. So, for most babies, rubbing a little oil, such as baby, mineral, or olive, into the scalp and simply combing out the flakes every day can help. In addition, you can shampoo twice a week with an antidandruff shampoo containing selenium or use one of the "baby"-oriented products designed for such a purpose. For babies with more skin involvement, a very small amount of low-dose steroid cream, such as 1% hydrocortisone, can be immensely helpful. However, your pediatrician should be involved in the decision to treat the condition with medication. Very rarely will a baby require any treatment with a prescription cream but more severe cases warrant a visit to the pediatrician. During daylight hours. No big rush.

## STEROID EFFECTS

Please limit the use of creams containing steroids to twice a day, for no more than seven days, and use sparingly. The steroid cream available over-the-counter is hydrocortisone but prescription creams containing steroids also end in -*one*, such as triamcinolone or betamethasone. Steroid creams should rarely, if ever, be used in the diaper area because they may be more absorbed into the body. There can be too much of a good thing and steroid creams, if used for a long time or in an overzealous manner, lead to thinning of the skin, changes in the pigment, and even problems with the natural steroids that control major things like blood sugar. However, when used as prescribed, these medications are very safe. And no, these are not the same steroids that weight lifters take.

Ringworm of the scalp occurs quite frequently in kids, particularly those of African descent. Anywhere on the body, ringworm looks like it says: a ring, which is usually slightly raised and scaly. Ringworm on the scalp, called tinea capitis, may appear more circular, with broken-off hairs and hair loss. Unfortunately, once this fungal infection gets into the hairline, it can be treated only with prescription medication by mouth. Creams will *not* work. The medication needs to get into the growing hairs to kill the infection. Occasionally a ringworm lesion of the scalp will cause a big immune system response. As a kid's immune system tries to attack the infection, the area can become large and swollen and even covered in white pus. This looks like a nasty bacterial infection, but in reality, antibiotics won't touch it because it's not an infection; it's all the white blood cells and other infection-fighting troopers swarming about. When this big, goopy mess happens, it is called a kerion, and can be treated with a steroid medication taken by mouth. Either way, if your little one gets a terrible-looking kerion, or has just plain old ringworm in the scalp, you will have to see your doctor. In the morning.

## Rashes on the Face

There are many rashes that begin on the face or scalp and can spread downward, and then there are rashes that are most commonly found on the face, although they can appear elsewhere.

Impetigo is a bacterial infection of the skin that causes honey-colored, crusted lesions, usually around the mouth and nose. These spots can look very crusty and gross and tend to spread, with smaller spots developing near the first one. Impetigo is very common in kids and is more common during the summer, although a child may become infected any time of year. Your doctor will need to prescribe antibiotics, either by mouth or in a cream, to treat this infection.

Petechiae are tiny red dots, the size of a pinhead. These are actually itty-bitty broken blood vessels that can occur from coughing (or screaming or vomiting) hard, but also may be an early sign of a more serious illness. Petechiae commonly occur on the cheeks and around the eyes, but if they travel south of the neck and appear anywhere else on the body, call your doctor. While petechiae on the body are frequently caused by harmless viral infections, your doctor will certainly want someone to have a look to make sure there is nothing else of significance happening.

A child who suddenly has bright red cheeks, sometimes accompanied by a fine, lacy rash all over the body, has the "slapped cheek" virus, otherwise known as fifth disease, or parvovirus. This particular virus is pretty common in kids and they seem to weather through it just fine, usually within a week. Any age can have a parvovirus infection, but older kids and teenagers may feel much more ill, with fever, aches, and swelling of the joints. It is important that pregnant women let their doctor know if they have been around a child with parvovirus, since this virus may, very rarely, cause problems in babies whose mothers weren't already immune to this particular bug. Good thing is, most of us already are. No need for panic.

## TRY SOME SOAP

Before you run your child out the door and to the doctor because of a worrisome spot or rash, humor me and try to wash it off. I'm not joking. I have removed more "chemical burns," "bruises," "petechiae," and "blue toes" with an alcohol swab than I care to remember. It's funny. But the parents always feel a little dumb. So just think back: Are those petechiae or was he playing with a blow pen?

Photodermatitis is a funny condition that happens when sunlight causes a chemical reaction in the skin if exposed to certain substances at the same time. Classically, lemons and limes do this, but so can celery, figs, parsnips, and dill. So if you let your baby suck on the limes from your Corona while at the beach, she's going to have a fantastic red ring around her mouth in the morning. This rash can occur anywhere on the body, but in kids it is seen most commonly on the face, since they are more likely to chew on a lemon than rub it on their arms. Don't worry about it. The discoloration may be red or brown in color and will gradually fade over the next several weeks to months. And keep your beer away from the baby.

And finally, Popsicle panniculitis is a condition that presents with firm, red-to-purple lumps in the cheeks. This is due to a baby sucking on very cold things, such as a frozen pacifier, teething ring, or, obviously, Popsicles, causing the fat in the cheeks to freeze and become inflamed. This will go away with time and there is nothing to worry about. However, a red and inflamed cheek could be due to an infection in the skin, so if your baby is otherwise ill, such as with fever, or the redness is only to one side of the mouth, let your doctor know.

## Rashes with Blisters

If one blister appears on your child's foot, he needs new shoes. But if bunches of blisters begin appearing in places, they are most likely due to an infection. Most infections that cause blisters are no big deal and don't need any treatment, but keep reading.

If your kid does develop a blister from his ill-fitting shoes, do *not* pop it. The fluid inside the blister protects the injured skin from both infection and further injury. Keep it covered and well padded to alleviate pain. Other than that, there is nothing you can do but wait and try a different pair of footwear.

***Chicken Pox.*** Chicken pox, or varicella, is a virus that classically gives small itchy blisters all over the body that are described as "dewdrops on rose petals." The blisters arrive in bunches, or "crops," and new ones can appear for several days. Most kids are immunized against the varicella virus, since it can be quite serious. However, if your baby is not yet one, she hasn't had this shot. Even with immunization, a child can still come down with chicken pox, but will have a much milder illness and isn't likely to be contagious. Some parents don't want to immunize their child against chicken pox because they think it is a normal childhood rite of passage. Be forewarned, before children in the United States began routinely receiving the varicella vaccine, hundreds of children and adults were hospitalized every year with severe infections that could even, rarely, be fatal.

## WHERE DID SHE GET IT?

Older folks may get a condition called shingles, caused by the chicken pox virus. After the initial illness, the virus stays in the body, and then years later, it may wake up in a nerve root, causing a terribly painful, blistery rash over just one area (on one side) of the body. This condition *is* contagious and may be where your peanut picked up her pox.

If you think your kid has chicken pox, call your pediatrician, although there isn't much to do for an otherwise healthy child other than to try to keep her happy with pain and fever control and itch management. If your kid is infected

## IF YOUR KID HAS THE POX

It is very, very important that anyone with an immune problem, cancer, or ill health; those who are elderly; and pregnant women who haven't been previously infected or immunized be told about your child's condition and avoid further contact until she is all better.

with chicken pox and has never been immunized against it, she is terribly contagious and will remain so until all the blisters are completely scabbed over, which may take two weeks.

If your child has the chicken pox and is becoming more ill or developing vomiting or difficulty breathing, call your doctor. Acting confused or complaining of a severe headache also warrants a phone call. Furthermore, if one spot begins to look infected, becoming redder, larger, and more painful, let your doctor know right away.

## TREATING THE POX

Good old-fashioned home remedies, such as oatmeal baths, might help to control the itching, as will over-the-counter antihistamines given by mouth. Fever and pain control will make your little chick feel a lot better. Age-appropriate doses of acetaminophen are good for this. Some physicians will advise against giving ibuprofen to kids with chicken pox because of its similarity to aspirin, which was linked to a severe illness in children after viral infections, particularly varicella infection.

*Big Blisters.* Bullous impetigo is another cause of blisters on the body, and can occur anywhere, most commonly in the diaper area. These blisters are much larger than the little chicken pox blisters and often quite red and may be full of yellow fluid or pus. You should let your doctor know about this rash, since it will require antibiotics. The younger your baby is, the more urgently you should contact your pediatrician, since the infection can, rarely, cause a bacterial infection in the bloodstream that can become quite serious. This more severe infection occurs most commonly in people with immature or weakened immune systems, such as little babies.

If your kid has such a rash and develops a fever, vomiting, or is otherwise not looking well, call your pediatrician.

Both hives and a condition called erythema multiforme can appear as large blisters, rather than spots. This presentation is far less common, but both conditions are generally quite harmless. You can read more about these conditions later in this chapter.

*Little Blisters.* Impetigo may also cause an infection of the body that does not cause large, fluid-filled blisters. This form of impetigo is called nonbullous impetigo, and is most commonly seen on the face. However, impetigo can occur anywhere and begins as a small blister, which then pops and forms a yellow, crusty spot. These spots will need treatment with an antibiotic cream or they will continue to spread.

Small blisters in groups, such as on the scalp or near the lip, may be caused by the herpes virus. As I've said, there are two types of herpes virus, the first being extremely common and causing simple cold sores in many adults. The second type is the one you are panicking about, but rest assured, most cases of herpes infection are *not* sexually transmitted. Either type of the herpes virus may cause symptoms in either place and both are very contagious. The first time someone has a herpes infection, he will feel much more ill than with a simple cold sore. The primary infection is often associated with more than one sore, which can coat the lips and around the mouth. More information on a herpes infection of the lips can be found in Chapter 5. Once you have the herpes virus, it lives in you forever and can act up periodically, causing an outbreak. We only worry about herpes because it causes pain and discomfort and because in some people, such as the very young or those with weakened immune systems, it can cause serious infection.

## UNDER THREE MONTHS

Any blistery-looking rash on a baby less than three months of age should absolutely be brought to your doctor's attention immediately. In small infants, herpes may present with small blisters at the scalp, where the monitor sat during labor. Herpes in small babies may cause serious illness and needs to be recognized and treated right away. This is also a very good reason why you shouldn't bite your baby's hangnails. The virus can be transmitted from your mouth to her fingers, even if you don't have a cold sore. Call your doctor if you are worried.

*Blisters on the Hands and Feet.* Tiny, white blisters appearing on the palms of the hands, the soles of the feet, and sometimes in the back of the throat or in the diaper area are due to the Coxsackie virus. This virus is commonly called hand, foot, and mouth disease, although I call it the hand, foot, mouth, and *butt* disease, because sometimes the blisters are in the diaper area and nowhere else. Coxsackie virus is very common in babies and little kids, occurring most frequently in the spring and summer, although anyone can get it at any time of year. Coxsackie infections are very commonly associated with high fevers, about 103°F or 104°F. The blisters actually reassure your doctor that the fever is due to a common virus. The spots will go away within about a week and don't need any treatment.

Scabies is another condition that may cause little blisters all over. Scabies is actually a skin infection caused by a little mite that gets under the skin and burrows around. Kids get it all the time and it is in no way a reflection of your child's hygiene or the cleanliness of your house. Classically, scabies causes intense itching and the little tunnels made by the

## FEVER REMINDER

Most rashes with blisters are caused by viruses, and most viruses cause fever. Try to remember that we aren't excited about the *height* of the fever, only the cause and how a kid is handling the illness, so you don't need to call your doctor just to report the fever if your kid is over three months and otherwise acting okay. Skip ahead to Chapter 10.

burrowing mites can be seen between the fingers and toes. However, in babies and young children, scabies may actually occur all over and not just between the digits. The rash may look like little blisters and the continuous scratching may cause scattered scabs and bumps. The little tunnels look like three little bumps right in a row, which is a big clue for scabies. Scabies is pretty contagious, especially among kids, so your doctor is probably going to want to treat the whole family with a prescription cream that is applied from the neck down and left on overnight. Even after treatment, the itching may continue although the rash should not continue to spread. An over-the-counter or prescription antihistamine is pretty helpful for kids with scabies. If the itching persists longer than a week or the rash seems to be getting worse, your doctor may choose to treat again in about seven days.

A not infrequent condition seen in children with their first herpes infection is herpetic whitlow. This is when the herpes virus causes an infection of the fingers. It's an easy scenario to imagine: toddler with cold sore, puts everything in his mouth, sucks on his fingers. The fingers become red, swollen, and covered in horrible white blisters. It looks absolutely terrible and your doctor will want to see him to make sure that it truly is a case of whitlow. Many people confuse a case of whitlow with a severe bacterial infection of the fingers, which can be an emergency, and it is important to make the distinction. However, unlike a bacterial infection, whitlow will not respond to antibiotics and heals up fine on its own. Just like with herpes infections of the lips, an antiviral medication may be helpful if started early, so be on the lookout for finger sores if your kid has a bad case of cold sores and is a finger sucker.

## Spots and Bumps

Random bumps and dots are rarely of concern. Some spots are permanent, such as moles, while others are temporary and some are due to infectious agents. If a spot has been there awhile, unless particularly large or interfering with daily life, such as a big mole on the bottom of the foot that makes walking difficult, you don't need a special appointment. Just let your doctor know at the next checkup. Otherwise don't be too worried.

*One Part of the Body.* An infection of the skin can be very tiny, like a pimple, or can cover a larger area, even several inches. When the infection is individual small spots, we will call this folliculitis. If the spots are yellow, crusty, and spreading, this would be indicative of impetigo, which is most commonly seen around the nose and mouth but can occur anywhere. Simple folliculitis will often go away with simple measures such as a little antibacterial soap scrub and possibly an antibiotic cream. If the spots become any bigger, an antibiotic cream, or occasionally medicine by mouth, is generally indicated. That said, knowing which spots are actually infectious and require treatment can be tricky, so let your doctor make the call.

Warmth and redness on the skin may indicate a bacterial infection, called cellulitis. We all have bacteria living on our skin and a tiny cut, or even a bug bite, can create a pathway through which these bacteria can enter the skin and set up camp. Cellulitis can cover a small area, the size of a coin, or can become quite large, stretching over part of an entire limb. When a child has such a skin infection, he will generally require antibiotics by mouth and should see his pediatrician soon. Rarely, a case of cellulitis can cause more serious illness, and a kid with symptoms such as fever or vomiting in the presence of skin infection should absolutely see a physician in an urgent fashion. If your kid is on antibiotics for a presumed cellulitis and seems to be worsening or develops new symptoms, call your doctor. We are seeing more and more infections that do not respond to our more common antibiotics and we need to get more creative when attacking some infections.

Not all infected spots and bumps are due to bacterial infections. Warts are fleshy little growths that are caused by viruses. Underneath the thick dry skin you can often see tiny

### IS IT AN INFECTION OR WHAT?

Many parents confuse a bug bite for a skin infection and vice versa. Many physicians also have trouble telling the difference. A bug bite is generally itchy, can cause swelling, and is usually pretty confined to one area. Pus does not drain from bug bites. Bug bites also get better within a day or two. Untreated skin infections, however, may grow larger over hours or days, are generally more tender and not itchy, and may be accompanied by other symptoms such as fever or vomiting. When in doubt, call your doctor.

## Permanent Ink

A good way to know for sure whether a possible skin infection is improving or spreading is to outline the rash with a permanent marker. We do this all the time in the hospital and it is a very helpful way of knowing if an infection is becoming worse and how quickly it is spreading. Your doctor will be very appreciative if your kid shows up with three different colors of marker that are dated and timed on his leg. It takes away the guesswork.

black dots. Those dots are the live part of the wart. Warts look nasty and parents hate them. The problem with warts is that they are extremely difficult to treat and will, eventually, go away on their own. If you are really fixated on curing your child's warts, speak to your pediatrician. There are over-the-counter treatments, prescription treatments, and all sorts of home remedies you can try, from banana peels to duct tape. Or you can just wait it out.

*All over the Body.* There are a couple of times when the appearance of a rash should make you take notice. As mentioned before, tiny broken blood vessels can occur quite easily on the face after screaming, violently coughing, or vomiting. These pinpoint little red dots are called petechiae and are nothing to worry about. When petechiae occur below the neck, however, you need to call your doctor. While a simple virus is the cause of most cases of petechiae on the body, a more severe infection or a problem with the blood's clotting system is, in rare cases, to blame. Since these are conditions that we don't want to miss, your pediatrician will want to hear from you right away. Larger red, blue, purple, or brown spots or bruises that appear all over the body also deserve immediate attention. These are called purpura, and are like a grown-up version of petechiae. Major infections or other causes of abnormal clotting of the blood could cause such bruising and you want to get right on that. A rash that looks like a severe sunburn but isn't is also something that should get you to call your doctor, particularly if your little one has a fever or is very irritable or ill appearing. As always, when in doubt, give your doc a ring.

> ## EMERGENCY!
>
> Any rash appearing below the neck that looks like bruising or a very bad sunburn (with or without blisters) requires an immediate phone call to your pediatrician.

As for the rest of the possible rashes covering the body, we don't generally get that excited. Some rashes are typically itchy in nature. Take, for example, hives, or urticaria, a common childhood rash. Hives are red bumps, occurring generally everywhere. They may take many shapes and be quite huge at times. The hallmark feature of hives is that the bumps move around. That is, they appear in one spot, fade over a period of time, and reappear in another spot. There might always be fifteen spots on your baby's belly, but not always in exactly the same location. Because the reaction is coming from the inside of the body (hence the moving spots), creams to treat the rash won't work. An antihistamine by mouth may help with the itching and discomfort. Be aware that once hives occur, they may come and go for a couple of weeks. As long as your kid is otherwise happy and not having any trouble breathing, there is nothing to worry about. Erythema multiforme is a rash that can look very similar to hives but the spots don't move. I mention it because a frustrated parent who had never heard of such a thing once accused me of "making it up." So now you've heard of it. Many different things can cause EM, which looks like big red targets all over the body. Unlike hives, the spots don't move. They will gradually turn darker and then fade over the next couple of weeks. No specific treatment is necessary. With either hives or erythema multiforme, if your kid doesn't seem to mind, you shouldn't either. However, if he is having swelling of the lips or face, difficulty breathing, or is acting more ill, call your pediatrician immediately.

## HIVES AREN'T JUST FOR HONEY

Parents are often surprised to learn that most cases of hives are *not* due to an allergic reaction. Viruses, changes in temperature, stress, medications, and "who the heck knows" are all common causes of hives. There's no point in killing yourself trying to figure out why.

Other rashes are commonly accompanied by a fever. Roseola is a terrible-looking pink or red, spotty rash that covers the whole body and is part of a classic viral syndrome. The spots can be as small as a pimple or bigger like a dime. This illness is most common in kids between six and twenty-four months old. After two to four days of high fever and no other symptoms, a terrific rash appears at the same time the fever goes away. Maybe your doctor was worried about the cause of the fever, depending on the age of your child, but the appearance of the rash alleviates any concern. Your little one is fine, needs no treatment, and you don't have to do a thing. Scarlet fever is a rash that can develop with certain strep throat infections. This rash is usually found all over the body but you might see it best on the chest, tummy, or back. It is typically red and very bumpy and feels like sandpaper. The typical signs of strep throat, such as fever, vomiting, or a sore throat, may be present. This rash is pretty classic and your doctor will recognize it right away. For more information on the infection that causes scarlet fever, go check out Chapter 5. Finally, a red rash all over the body that is accompanied by a very high fever for several days may be due to Kawasaki's disease. This condition can be difficult to diagnose and does require treatment to prevent long-term complications. However, a rash and a fever are definitely not the only symptoms (check out Chapter 10), and it is pretty rare. Call your pediatrician if you are worried.

## PEELING

After certain infections, classically scarlet fever or Kawasaki's disease, a child's skin may peel, particularly over the hands, feet, and in the diaper area. The peeling is completely normal but looks mighty impressive. Don't worry about it.

Some kids will develop a rash that looks like red, purple, or brown spots over the backs of their arms, legs, and buttocks. The rash may follow a viral illness or be due to some other agent that has revved up the immune system. This condition is called Henoch-Schönlein purpura, or HSP, and is a form of vasculitis, or inflammation of the blood vessels. HSP most commonly affects kids between the ages of two and eleven and can also cause pain and inflammation of the joints, such as the elbows or knees. HSP usually goes away all by itself over a couple of weeks and most often requires no treatment. However, some kids will develop kidney or intestinal problems, so belly pain, dark urine, or blood in the stool should prompt a quick middle-of-the-night call to your pediatrician.

### It's Not Really a Spot or a Dot but . . .

And finally, what if you can't really categorize what is happening by location, or because it isn't really a rash but maybe it is and her skin is sort of dry but maybe not and on you go?

*Dry Skin.* Dry skin may occur all over, or it may occur in patches. Sometimes dry itchy skin is due to an allergy or irritation from a lotion or other substance. These conditions are called allergic and contact dermatitis. Check out Chapter 11. Dry skin everywhere may be simply dry skin, or it may become a more serious condition called eczema. Dry skin in patches may also be eczema, but a few other conditions, such as psoriasis, can cause thick dry skin. Ask your doctor if you aren't sure.

Eczema is a dry, flaky, itchy rash that occurs commonly in allergic little kids. The best description I've ever heard is that this is the "itch that rashes." In other words, extremely itchy skin becomes red and inflamed in response to scratching, and can become very flaky and dry, with gradual scarring and thickening. Thus, the key to treating eczema is to avoid the scratching. Since babies and small children tend to ignore my sage advice, what you can do to help her is to try to keep the skin from itching. Moisture is the key. Contrary to popular belief, taking a bath won't dry out the skin. Very frequent, hot baths not followed by moisturizing *can* dry your skin. But since we are waterproof, the only way your outer layer of skin can become wetter is by putting water on it. Think about it: If we weren't waterproof, we'd be leaking everywhere. You couldn't wear silk or suede. It would be very messy. So get the skin wet. Then you've got to seal that water in. So don't rub her dry. Let her play in the water until she's nice and wrinkly, then pull her out and pat her *just enough* to keep from dripping water all over the floor. Follow this with the thickest coat of the greasiest thing you can find. It can be expensive or cheap. Crisco, petroleum jelly, olive oil. They all work. Sally should slip out of your hands like a greased pig. Then dress her in something warm and soft and not itchy. Do this a couple of times a week, with heavy moisturizing a couple of times a day, and for most mild cases of eczema, you should see an improvement. Basically, she should never feel dry to you. Moisturize. Moisturize. Moisturize.

If your doctor has given you a prescription for a steroid or other type of eczema cream, apply the cream as directed just *before* the moisturizer and only to the dry areas, trying to avoid the normal skin. Some babies will have more severe disease, despite your best efforts, and will need more aggressive management and possibly referral to a dermatologist, or skin specialist.

**Really Pale Kids.** Some babies will have a fine, lacy appearance to their skin. It may appear blotchy at times and worsen with exposure to cold air. This is completely normal and means absolutely nothing.

A very pale-appearing infant who is otherwise happy and vigorous likely just has porcelain-perfect skin and would be lucky to stay that way (sunscreen, hint hint!). However, extremely pale skin may be a sign of anemia (low hemoglobin or red blood cells). If the baby appears particularly pale next to your own skin, especially if she seems to be less active or sleepier than other babies or has trouble feeding, please let your pediatrician know.

There is a group of special little tykes who deserve mention here. They are the Milk Babies. Cow's milk is a great source of fat and calcium and protein and vitamin D and all that. But it was actually intended for consumption by baby cows. Thus, cow's milk can cause irritation of our intestines and microscopic bleeding. In other words, you won't see blood in your stool, but you are losing small amounts of it anyway. Add this to the fact that cow's milk is a very poor source of iron, and you can see how kiddos who drink large amounts of regular cow's milk may be at risk for anemia. Please note that infant formula made from cow's milk is fortified with extra iron, and is designed for babies, so we are talking about regular cow's milk only, not baby formula.

Most babies switch from formula to regular milk at one year of age. Unfortunately, many of them really, really like their milk. And since it's so good for us, many parents let

## COW'S MILK IS FOR BABY COWS

How much milk should your kid drink? Naturally, babies under one year of age will get the majority of their calories and nutrition from either breastmilk or formula. Older babies and toddlers generally switch to regular milk until about age two, when they can move on to whatever the family prefers. Two dairy servings a day is appropriate for a preschooler, which means limiting her to sixteen to twenty-four ounces of milk (or the equivalent in yogurt, cheese, or other dairy products). This will give her a good dose of calcium, fat, and protein without the side effects that can occur from too much milk, such as constipation and anemia.

them drink as much as they want. A few kids develop such a fantastic milk habit that they actually receive the majority of their calories from milk, meaning that they replace other sources of iron in their diets. All this can make for a very chubby (because milk is full of calories), very pale (because he has very low iron and develops anemia) toddler. The hemoglobin levels in these kids can become dangerously, frighteningly low, requiring hospitalization and sometimes blood transfusions. Because the anemia develops so slowly, these children display very few signs of anemia, other than being extremely pale and maybe having a slightly higher-than-normal heart rate. In other words: All things are good, in moderation.

# you give me fever!

Fever in a newborn *is* an emergency. But the older a child gets, the less and less exciting fever becomes. Fever is the body's way of pumping up your immune system, calling in the troops, and attacking whatever is making you feel punky and miserable. The cause of the fever is generally considered to be of greater importance than the fever itself. Parents focus a lot of energy on the specific height of the fever. Everyone is worried that if the fever creeps up to a terribly "dangerous" height, the baby's brain is going to boil and he'll die. He won't boil his brain. I promise. But sometimes a fever does warrant a phone call to the pediatrician and sometimes it is nothing to worry about. This chapter will explain the difference between a fever that is concerning and one that is nothing to fear.

## Fever Defined and Measured

### What Is a Fever?

A normal body temperature is 98.6°F. This number is an average, so some people may run a degree higher or lower. A normal temperature is the optimal warmth for our blood to flow smoothly, our brain to use oxygen, and all our parts and pieces to operate as intended. Being in a very warm or cold environment may affect our body temperature, as can exercise and wearing many layers of clothing. We care about changes in

## DON'T MAKE ME SAY IT AGAIN

Fever is only a symptom, not something to fear. It isn't harmful. Only the things that cause a fever can hurt a child. Not the fever itself.

temperature because a higher or lower temperature may indicate an infection or other problem with our body's temperature regulation center.

A fever is a temperature above the range of normal body temperatures and often indicates an infection of some type. For babies and children, a temperature of 100.4°F (38°C) is considered a fever. Most fevers are caused by viral infections and the specific number of degrees is not important. However, there are times when we do want to know a child's exact temperature. Keep reading.

## How to Measure a Temperature

Unfortunately, kissing your little pumpkin's forehead and telling me he has a temperature won't cut the mustard. "Feel-

## HOW HIGH IS TOO HIGH?

I know that Grandma's going to have a heart attack now, but I must insist that there is no such thing as a fever that is too high. Your brain has a fever center, which generates a fever in response to infection. The fever center is limited when it comes to how high a fever can be. The highest a fever can go is really about 106° to 107°F. A body temperature higher than this usually means that another force is at work, such as being left inside a very hot car on a summer day and being "cooked" from the outside. Or the thermometer is broken.

FEAR OF FEVER

*Fever phobia* is the term that those of us "in the know" use to describe the fear that parents have of fever in babies and children. Fever is not dangerous and needs to be controlled only if causing symptoms, such as feeling really cruddy.

ing hot" to a parent is a very unreliable method of detecting a fever, so we need to find another way for you to measure your kid's temperature.

The most common way to measure temperature in babies is with a rectal thermometer, and it is the method most commonly preferred by many medical professionals, especially for small babies. A digital thermometer is probably what you have at home, since the old-fashioned mercury ones not only were difficult to read, but could be dangerous if broken open. Put a little bit of petroleum jelly on the tip, insert the thermometer gently into the rectum until you can't see the metal anymore (about a half inch), and wait until it beeps. The number you see is the rectal temperature.

Many parents shy away from rectal thermometers, especially as their child gets a bit older and begins to find the whole process rather distasteful. Taking a temperature by mouth in a baby or small child is nearly impossible, so placing the thermometer firmly in the armpit, or axilla, will give a pretty good, although not perfect, estimation of a child's temperature, which we call the axillary temperature.

Ear thermometers, temperature-taking pacifiers, and fancy little strips across the forehead are all alternative means of measuring temperature marketed toward parents. Although some are not as accurate as others, these products are all easy to use and seemingly less noxious. So, feel free to buy and use these products. If you decide you need to call your doctor because your child is either very young or has other concerning symptoms, just be sure to tell him both the temperature *and* what type of thermometer you used.

## CALCULATING A "TRUE" TEMPERATURE

Do *not* start adding numbers to the temperature to try to "equal" a rectal temperature. Yes, there may be a slight difference between a rectal and an axillary, oral, or ear temperature. But your doctor really wants to know both the number you saw and how the temperature was taken. Say, "Hi, Doc, little Henry has a temp of 102 on the ear thermometer." Otherwise things can get mighty confusing.

## Fever by Age

Fever in a baby or child is one of the few conditions handled differently by age. The younger the baby, the more likely we are to test for infections of the blood, urine, and nervous system, even without evidence of infection on exam. Once a baby is older and the immune system is more mature, accompanying signs and symptoms, as well as the duration of the illness, become more important. So, let's break this down first by age group. Plow ahead.

### Newborn: Zero to Twenty-eight Days

Pay close attention. This is the only time that I will refer to fever as an emergency. Fever is a normal physiologic response to infection. But newborns aren't normal creatures. Fever in a newborn is a whole different thing from fever in nearly everyone else. Their immune systems are immature and highly ineffective. What's more, fever in a very young infant may signal an infection that was acquired during birth or soon thereafter. These infections are in no way a reflection of Mom's hygiene or the cleanliness of the hospital. They are specific to newborn infants and can occur regardless of race, age, or socioeconomic status. It also doesn't matter to me if your three-week-old is the size of a six-month-old. It's age, not size, that matters.

## WHEN TO CALL WITHOUT READING FURTHER

The rules are very straightforward. An infant under one month with a fever of 100.4°F (38.0°C) or higher sees the doctor. Period. No discussion. As a general rule, a baby under twenty-eight days of age with a fever is going to the emergency room. Many infants between one and three months should also be seen in either the ER or the doctor's office, and you definitely should be calling your pediatrician.

What happens when a newborn is seen for a fever is subject to your doctor's experience, training, and style. You can expect that laboratory testing will be done, including examination of the blood, urine, and spinal fluid. A couple of days in the hospital waiting for the final results of all the tests is the norm. For me, this is a no-brainer. There is no art to the practice of medicine when it comes to a newborn with a fever.

Perhaps it seems a bit aggressive or mean of us to treat all newborns with a fever the same way. I guarantee that you don't like the idea of uncomfortable or possibly painful tests being performed on your sweet and defenseless baby. We all understand that and we don't like it any more than you do. But again, our job is to think of the worst and try to prevent that from happening. A couple of days in the hospital are no one's idea of fun. But we want your baby alive and well at the end of the day.

## How Scary Is a Spinal Tap?

If a baby or child comes to the ER and we are worried about meningitis, a lumbar puncture, or spinal tap, will be performed. Many parents freak out about this, but it is something we do all the time (even in itty-bitty babies) and with good reason: The complications of meningitis include blindness, deafness, developmental delay, and even death. For a better understanding of what a spinal tap actually means for a baby, see Chapter 15.

## One Month to Three Months

Fever in a newborn is a no-brainer. Urine, blood, spinal tap, IV, antibiotics, stay in the hospital for two to three days. No discussion. Babies are sneaky, especially the very young ones. Not only do they have silly baby immune systems, but they also like to hide all signs of serious disease from us until things have become dire. As a baby gets older, our paranoia begins to lessen. Now, logic would tell us that a baby who is twenty-nine days old is not *so* different from a twenty-eight-day-old. Therefore, for babies between four and eight weeks of age, management of fever is largely dependent on individual practices but is pretty similar to the management of newborns. Most physicians will continue to do a thorough evaluation on smaller infants although some babies may be sent home, with or without antibiotics, and followed very closely. We know that the vast majority of babies with fever simply have a viral illness. So, as a baby gets a bit older (six to eight weeks), some doctors will forgo some of the testing if everything else looks normal. From this point until twelve weeks of age, most of us will check blood and urine to start, with a spinal tap added later if there are any concerns. Naturally, if the baby looks ill, or there are concerning features to the history, your doctor will (and should!) become more aggressive, opting to include all testing and possibly admission to the hospital for antibiotics and/or observation. For babies under twelve weeks who are sent home after being evaluated for fever, some may be given a twenty-four-hour antibiotic shot, and will need to be seen daily for repeat injections until all the "cultures" (forty-eight to seventy-two hours) come back as negative.

Therefore, if your baby is younger than three months and has a fever over 100.4°F, call your doctor. She may decide to see you that day or send you to the ER, depending on what else is going on. Just be prepared that the younger the infant, the more likely it is that we will want to perform certain tests. Know that, as frightening as that may be, we do it all the time and with very good reason. You don't want to take any chances with your precious little sweet pea, do you?

## Three Months to Three Years

After twelve weeks, most babies are no longer in danger from the serious infections that can affect newborns. By the time your little one is three months old, chances are that any illness she acquires will be the same one you've got. Her sister comes home from preschool covered in germs, proceeds to lavish them all over you and her baby sister, and seven to ten days later you find yourself blowing your nose while simultaneously bulb-suctioning Cindy's. That said, pediatrics is a bit like veterinary medicine. Babies and very young children can't tell us what hurts or how they are feeling. The reason for a fever may be less clear. When an infant has a fever, and no source for the fever (such as a viral rash or an ear infection) can be found on examination, the decision to do further testing will depend on the time of year, the history, who else is sick at home, how closely you can follow up with your doctor, and a host of other factors, not the least of which is the particular practice of the physician you are seeing. For many years, guidelines regarding the evaluation and management of fever recognized children between three and thirty-six months of age as a separate entity from older children. The reason for this was that this group of kids had a slightly higher risk of acquiring certain types of infections. Many children were poked and prodded while their parents developed a falsely heightened sense of fear about fever. If you have an older child who was seen for "fever" and had a lot of tests and shots, you think I'm crazy for telling you not to worry about his sibling. Fortunately, times have changed. About a decade ago, children in the United States began routinely receiving the pneumococcal vaccine, also known as the "ear infection shot." Pneumococcus was one of the bugs that we used to worry about in babies. Since this risk was already really tiny, a further reduction in infections made us all feel a lot better about fever in young kids who have been properly immunized. Nowadays physicians are doing a lot less poking, prodding, and sticking of little kids with fever because we know that, in the absence of concerning signs or symptoms, the vast majority will have a viral illness. In other words, most kids need no treatment. I know what you want is an absolute. You want to be 100 percent sure that your child isn't the one in a million with a serious infection. Unfortunately, I can't give you that. Fever is so very common and is not in and of itself harmful. It is your job (and ours) to watch your kid closely to make sure he isn't developing signs of a more serious illness. You know your baby best, far better than any laboratory test.

## DOES A FEVER REQUIRE ANTIBIOTICS?

The absolute number one cause for a fever in a little one is a virus. Antibiotics can't touch a virus. Nothing can, except time, patience, and tender loving care. The inappropriate use of antibiotics in kids who don't need them can have significant consequences, such as the development of an allergy or resistance to the particular medication. Both of these mean that the antibiotic choices available to your doctor if your child *does* develop a bacterial infection become more limited and difficult.

So, if your little one is being evaluated for fever, there are several things that may happen. Nothing. Blood tests. Urine tests. Spinal tap. Chest X-rays. Antibiotics. No antibiotics. Hospital stay. Home with a sticker. There is no way to generalize what should be done for all babies and children with a fever. The only absolute is that fever makes us feel yucky. When our fever is high, we are mopey and cranky and listless and miserable. *However*, when a kid's fever comes down, he should be a bit more playful and acting more like himself. It is not unusual to be very listless or even to seem to have trouble breathing when a baby has a fever. *But* I don't care what he looks like when his fever is 102°F. I care about what he looks like when it has come back down. A child who is still listless, seems to have trouble breathing, is very cranky, refuses to eat or drink, or acts very irritable or sleepy, even after his temperature has dropped, is a kid that concerns me.

## How Important Is the Fever?

For a kid over three months of age and in generally good health, the presence or height of a fever is far less important than how she is acting. Bringing the fever down will let you see just how sick she really feels. Still acting like a lump when her temperature is normal is a sign that your doctor should be involved.

Some folks argue that we shouldn't even be treating fever, since it's our body's way of kicking our immune system in the pants and fighting off what ails us. However, fever makes all of us feel terrible and it is difficult to know if a baby is truly ill when his fever is making him so unhappy. So, if your kid is boiling away at 104°F but is happy and smiley and drinking and playing, you don't have to do a thing. If he's acting like a miserable bump on the sofa, give him an appropriate dose of acetaminophen or ibuprofen and wait an hour. If he all of a sudden perks up and looks a bit better, you can relax because it's likely to be nothing serious. But if his fever comes down and he still looks very sick, call your pediatrician immediately.

## Three Years and Beyond

Just like kids over three months, the vast, vast majority of children with a fever have a viral illness. If your kid is otherwise healthy, fever is not an emergency. Expect him to feel like garbage. As your brain tells your body to increase its temperature, lots of muscles start working and contracting to make heat. This can give us the shakes and chills, and make us achy and miserable. A fever can make every bone in the body hurt. As a child becomes old enough to verbalize this, she may complain of a head- or bellyache, or pain in her arms or legs. While it isn't necessary to treat the fever per se, it is okay to treat the aches and misery. Load him up with appropriate doses of your fever reducer of choice, get some soup, and turn on the telly.

If your child is still complaining of pain in the head or belly after the fever has come back down, if she refuses to move or complains of neck pain, or if she is having trouble breathing or acting more ill, call your pediatrician. All of these symptoms may occur *with* fever, but we want them to resolve when the fever comes down. As I've said before, I don't care what a kid looks like when his fever is 104°F; I care only about what he looks like when it is 99°F.

## Managing the Fever

There are two main over-the-counter medicines for pain and fever that are approved for use in infants and children. Acetaminophen, the main ingredient in Tylenol, is a safe and effective medication for infants and children of all ages. The proper dosing is 15 milligrams per kilogram of body weight, given every four to six hours. Of course, how many milligrams are in a teaspoon or a dropper will vary based upon the formulation. For example, infant Tylenol is much more concentrated than the children's formulation, so giving a teaspoon of infant drops could seriously hurt a child who is the right size for a teaspoon of the children's formulation. Your

## TREATING THE FEVER

Remember, there is no absolute reason to treat a fever. Fever is a natural response to infection and helps to boost our immune system. However, fever does make us feel miserable, increases our heart rate, makes us more likely to become dehydrated, and can make some children have difficulty breathing. A child who is not well appearing might benefit from fever reduction so you can tell if his symptoms are a result of the fever or his underlying illness. Call your doctor before treating a fever in a baby less than three months old.

doctor's office can help you figure out the appropriate dose for your child's weight and age; the dosing on the package label is often lower than optimal and may be inappropriate if your baby is particularly beefy or rather petite.

Acetaminophen has been associated with liver damage in people who take too high a dose, or have liver disease or drink excessive amounts of alcohol. While your infant is (hopefully!) not mixing grape Tylenol and vodka, an overdose can occur if the wrong dose is inadvertently administered, or if a baby is receiving two types of medication that both contain acetaminophen. If you have any concern that your child may have received too much medicine, call your pediatrician immediately!

Ibuprofen is the other commonly recommended medicine for pain and fever in infants and children. It is properly dosed at 10 milligrams per kilogram of body weight, every six to eight hours. But as with acetaminophen, the concentration of ibuprofen formulations will vary, and it is best to ask your doctor for help figuring out the appropriate dosages.

Ibuprofen is less dangerous than acetaminophen in small overdoses, but can cause stomach pain and rarely bleeding, even in normal amounts. In addition, ibuprofen is *not* yet approved for infants under six months of age. While many physicians will use it, the packaging will suggest that it is best reserved for home use in infants older than six months. Ibuprofen does have the added benefit of being an *anti-inflammatory*, meaning that it is good for treating not only pain, but also inflammation, or swelling, which can accompany injuries and other conditions, making it a better choice in certain situations. Your doctor can help you decide whether ibuprofen confers any advantage over acetaminophen for whatever is ailing your precious little bug.

## WHY IS IT CALLED BABY ASPIRIN?

Aspirin is routinely *not* recommended for infants or children. Aspirin has been associated with the development of Reye's syndrome in children, a condition that causes inflammation of the brain and liver. Unless there is a specific condition for which aspirin is recommended, baby aspirin is best left to Grandpa's healthy heart regimen! "Grandpa aspirin" would actually be a better name for it.

As for other means of treating a fever, do *not* use alcohol baths or ice baths. The use of rubbing alcohol to increase cooling of the skin has been associated with severe poisonings in small children who have absorbed the alcohol through their skin. Stripping him naked and running a fan over him or placing him in a cold bath are not only unnecessary, but may make things worse. Your body raises its temperature, in part, by contracting all the muscles of the skin and body. Plunging into an ice bath will make a child shiver and shake, which might actually *raise* his temperature! Plus, it's mean.

## Febrile Seizures

I know about now you are thinking: But what about those kids who have a fever so high that they go into convulsions? That's what Grandma is *really* warning me about! Well, I'm going to quell your fears. A febrile seizure is a seizure (or convulsions) that occurs with a fever. Contrary to popular belief, these seizures don't happen because the fever was so high that it damaged the brain. In about 2 to 4 percent of all kids (mostly between six months and six years of age), a sudden rise in body temperature can trigger a seizure. Most of the time the seizure is less than five minutes long and involves the whole body. Of course, this is incredibly scary and I don't blame parents for panicking. However, by the time a parent has called 911, the seizure has almost always stopped, and by the time the ambulance arrives at the emergency room, the kid is back to his happy, playful self.

### HE'S BOILED HIS BRAIN

Febrile seizures are *not* the result of a high fever "cooking" a child's brain. They are a natural, albeit impressive, response to the *rise* in temperature in a small percentage of children. In other words, it's not the fever of 105°F that will cause a seizure; it is the sudden spike in temperature from normal to high.

The thing that is tough about febrile seizures is that we have no way of knowing *which* kid will have one and *if* he'll ever have another! As a general rule, kids who come from families with a history of febrile seizures are at slightly higher risk. Many children who have one febrile seizure never have another, while others go into convulsions every time they are sick. This doesn't mean anything bad and doesn't worry us as physicians, but is a very scary thing for parents.

Some doctors will recommend that a child who has had a febrile seizure take medicine for fever around the clock, even alternating acetaminophen and ibuprofen every three to four hours. Of note, this practice has *never* been shown to be effective at preventing febrile seizures *and* has also not been proven to be an entirely safe practice. Giving both drugs around the clock does run the risk of exceeding the recommended safe dosage in a twenty-four-hour period. So speak to your doctor about the risk of future seizures and whether giving medication in an attempt to prevent a seizure is the right thing for your child.

If a child has one febrile seizure in a twenty-four-hour period, returns to normal, and otherwise looks well, not to worry. However, seizures with fever may rarely indicate a more serious problem, such as an infection in the fluid around the brain, called meningitis. Having more than one seizure, seizures that last longer than fifteen minutes, ones that

## THE REALLY YOUNG AND SEIZING FEBRILE CHILD

It is often recommended that strong consideration be given to performing a lumbar puncture, or spinal tap, in infants younger than twelve months who have a febrile seizure, especially if they are at all ill appearing. Febrile seizures are much less common in this age group and may be a sign of meningitis.

involve only part of the body (a focal seizure), or a failure to return to normal after the seizure are all signs that a febrile seizure may actually be something different and warrants further investigation.

## Prolonged Fever

How long can a child have a fever before we start to worry? Honestly, quite a long time. Most viral illnesses will last seven to ten days, sometimes up to two weeks. Since we know that most kids with fever have a virus, there is often little reason for concern if a child has fever for several days. With most viral illnesses, fever will be present for the first three to five days of the illness, then gradually disappear. A fever that lasts a few days longer or returns is most commonly still just the virus at work. On the other hand, there are some conditions where a prolonged or recurrent fever is of concern. So, how do you know the difference?

A fever that is present for a few days, resolves, and then returns again is most probably due to an entirely new illness. Kids who are around other children, such as those who attend daycare or come from large, extended families, are going to be exposed to a lot of germs. Children have, on average, about ten colds a year. This means a cold, and probably a fever, most months. Viruses don't pay attention to any scheduled timetable; one might just ride in on the tail of another.

On the other hand, a fever that resolves and then recurs and is accompanied by new and different symptoms, such as a worsening cough or ear pain, might be due to a secondary infection. This means that an infection, such as a cold, has created circumstances that are favorable for the arrival of a second infection. For example, a cold makes the tubes that drain fluid from the inner ear (the Eustachian tubes) puffy and swollen. When the fluid can't drain normally, bacteria may begin to grow and an ear infection develops. Therefore, new symptoms or worsening of an illness in a child who appeared to be on the mend a day ago would absolutely warrant a call to his doctor's office.

What about fever that never ends? Certainly we begin to look a little harder for the source of a fever when we hear that it has lasted longer than usual. It is important to tell your doctor how many days a fever has been present. However, let's be very clear on something. A kid who had a fever for three days, then didn't for two days, and then had a fever again for three days has *not* had a fever for eight days. Remember, he's probably had one cold followed by another. This is very different from a true fever for eight days. Also, it is important to distinguish between *true* fever, meaning over 100.4°F, and "feeling warm" or a temperature of 100°F. A prolonged fever is *not* eight days of a 99° to 100°F "fever." So now that we have that straight, if you are worried that your child truly has a fever that is continuing for longer than normal, please do let your doctor know.

One condition that must be mentioned here is Kawasaki's disease. This is a condition that occurs mostly in toddlers and is classically characterized by a fever more than five days in duration. The fevers are usually quite high (103° to 104°F) and accompanied by other, variable symptoms. Other signs of Kawasaki's disease include very red eyes, red lips and tongue, and a rash all over the body. Children with Kawasaki's disease tend to be irritable little buggers! They are just not happy campers. Unfortunately, Kawasaki's disease can cause abnormal ballooning of the arteries around the heart if it isn't recognized and treated early. Fortunately, it is pretty rare. There is no one test for Kawasaki's disease, so the diagnosis is made by looking at the whole child, checking a few lab tests, and deciding on whether it all fits. Once we think a kid might have this particular illness, an intravenous medication is started that resolves the fever within twenty-four hours. The earlier we start treatment, the less likely there will be any damage to the heart. Therefore, a fever does *not* have to last five days before a diagnosis is made and medication started. That said, just the fever, without any of the other signs of Kawasaki's disease, is *not* enough to start treatment, so don't panic when your child has a high fever for four days but otherwise looks well. If, however, you think that something unusual is going on, give your pediatrician a call.

# allergies, bites, and stings

In some ways it seems odd to include food allergies and animal bites in the same chapter. On the other hand, plenty of bites, stings, or animal contacts can imitate or cause allergic reactions. Is that blood in his poop an allergy to his formula or because he kissed the dog on the mouth? So I guess in a way, allergic reactions and interspecies interactions belong in the same place. Let's talk about allergies to food, the world, and medication, and about bites and stings from all kinds of creatures, as well as about making sure that any animals brought into the home don't cause your little one any undue harm.

## Allergic Reactions

### What Are They and Why?

Allergies aren't something that we are normally born with, yet some of us go on to develop horrible allergies while others seem to be allergic to nothing. I, unfortunately, was one of those gooby kids who carried her own dessert to birthday parties and saw her allergist twice a week for shots.

A simple allergic reaction usually involves just one part of your body: a runny itchy face (eyes and nose); an itchy rash (skin); vomiting, diarrhea, or bloody stools (the digestive tract); etc. In babies, allergies may present slightly differently than in older kids and adults, and the exact cause can be difficult to pinpoint. In really young kids, other than in cases of allergic colitis, a rash is the most common form of an allergic reaction. A rash may result from direct contact with something (such as a cream) or from a general exposure to an allergen. Eczema is the rash classically seen in allergic people. Hives are another rash that people want to blame on an allergic reaction. More information on both of these rashes can be found in Chapter 9.

## ⋺││!

A severe allergic reaction, called anaphylaxis, may cause swelling of the lips and tongue, difficulty breathing, vomiting, or passing out. Seek medical attention immediately if your child seems to be having more than a simple allergic reaction. Call 911.

Some kids will have a more significant allergic reaction that can cause symptoms such as difficulty breathing or swelling of the lips and tongue. These reactions are taken quite seriously, and if your kid has had such an experience, she's probably already seen a physician about it. The doctor may have given your child a prescription for an epinephrine injection, an EpiPen, to have for the initial treatment of a severe reaction. Since treatment with adrenaline, or epinephrine, in the first few minutes of a severe reaction may be lifesaving, it is important both to understand how to use the device and to have it always with you. Please remember, urgent medical treatment is imperative after using an EpiPen.

911!

If your kid has an EpiPen, or other auto-injecting epinephrine device, know how to use it. When you pull off the gray safety cap, make sure your fingers don't go near the black end of the device. Then slam it down against his thigh muscle. Through the clothes is fine. And I mean slam. The needle is triggered by a forceful motion and is strong enough to go through denim if necessary. Hold the unit in place for at least ten seconds. Then call 911 or get to the nearest ER. If you have one, you should use your second EpiPen in five minutes if there are still significant symptoms or if symptoms return before finding medical attention.

If your baby is unconscious, blue, or having trouble breathing, call 911 for immediate attention.

## Food Allergies

While rare in the very young infant, older infants may develop allergies to certain foods. Figuring out which foods are the exact offenders may be difficult. For example, a kid might be labeled "allergic" to tomatoes when the true allergen is a tiny bit of coriander maybe not even listed on the ingredients label of the sauce. An allergist may need to help decide whether a reaction actually is an allergy and to which

911!

If a kid develops swelling around the lips or tongue, a raspy voice, difficulty breathing, or seems very ill, this is an emergency and you should call 911.

## THE OFFENDERS

Any kid can be allergic to any food, but 90 percent of all food allergies are to peanuts, tree nuts (such as walnuts and cashews), milk, eggs, wheat, soy, fish, and shellfish. When seeing a kid for a first-time severe allergic reaction, I will often advise parents to avoid not only the suspected offender, but also peanuts and tree nuts (which are notorious for causing severe reactions), until seen by an allergist. Fantastic food allergy information can be found at www.foodallergy.org.

foods little Gordon is allergic. Treatment generally consists of avoiding the offending chow. Many parents think their kid has an "allergy" because he spits up. Spitting up, or reflux, is very rarely due to a true allergy. A few kids may be more sensitive to certain things in Mom's diet or the formula, but for the vast majority of babies, the answer is simply that she's a spitter. Crying, or colic, is also unlikely to be due to an "allergy" in little babies, although spending hours eliminating this or that from her diet might provide some distraction until she has a more mature brain and shuts up.

## BABY SHOTS

Although there were concerns in the past, studies have shown that the MMR (measles, mumps, and rubella) vaccine can be safely given to kids with egg allergies. The flu vaccine, however, is made using eggs and may not be safe for all kids with an allergy to eggs. Your doctor or allergist can perform a sensitivity test to decide whether this important vaccine can be safely administered.

## Medication Allergies

True allergies to medicines are pretty rare. Vomiting after taking a certain medication or developing a rash after starting an antibiotic is rarely due to a real allergy. For example, many viral illnesses will give a child a rash. If you start an antibiotic and then develop a rash, who is to say that the rash wouldn't have been there anyway? Of the people who believe they are allergic to penicillin, less than 2 percent of them have a true allergy when tested at a doctor's office. Moreover, allergies do run in families, but not necessarily allergies to the same drugs. So, if Mom is allergic to penicillin, it isn't a given that the kid will be. If he is, it's because he's just an allergic sort of child. So, it is important to watch your baby closely after giving her any medication, but be aware that many "reactions" are either normal side effects or coincidental. Diarrhea is a normal side effect of antibiotics, and most cases of rash or hives are actually unrelated to the medicine. Speak with your pediatrician if you have any concerns that your child is reacting poorly to a medication.

> **911!**
>
> If your child develops swelling of the face, difficulty breathing, or any other signs that she is truly ill after taking anything, call 911 without delay.

If you think your kid has a true medication allergy, it might be worth having her tested by an allergist. A presumed allergy may force physicians to unnecessarily choose alternative antibiotics that are less than ideal for the condition needing treatment.

## WHAT ABOUT "PENICILLIN-LIKE" ANTIBIOTICS?

Many people with a "penicillin" allergy believe that they can't take antibiotics from the cephalosporin family either, but this has been shown to be untrue. A person with a true penicillin allergy is just as likely to react to a cephalosporin as to any other antibiotic because the person is just prone to allergies. Anyone who has had an anaphylactic reaction to *any* antibiotic should be closely monitored for an allergic reaction when receiving any new medication.

## Other Allergic Rashes

If your kid smears herself with your fancy face cream and develops a rash, the rash may be an allergy or may simply be the result of contact with an irritating substance. This type of rash is called allergic or contact dermatitis. *Dermatitis* is just a fancy word for *rash*. Allergic and contact dermatitis look the same and are generally red, itchy, and bumpy. Over long periods of time the skin can become thickened or change in pigment, becoming either lighter or darker. Honestly, it doesn't really matter a whole lot whether the rash is from an irritant or an allergy since the treatment is the same. Avoid contact with the offender. If the rash is really itchy or inflamed, your doctor can prescribe some mild steroid cream for a few days to quiet things down. An antihistamine by mouth in an age- and size-appropriate dose will also help with the itching.

One specific type of allergic dermatitis is a nickel allergy. Nickel is a metal that can be found in accessories, such as snaps and earrings. Kids with a nickel sensitivity may develop a chronic round rash on their bellies, right where the snap from their pants rubs. Little girls with pierced ears may have red, scaly, or thickened earlobes. There is nothing to do if your little one develops an allergy to nickel other than to avoid it. Buy nickel-free jewelry and try covering the inside of the snap with some duct tape. As long as the metal isn't directly in contact with the skin, it will be fine. Some kids will outgrow this allergy and others have it for the rest of their lives. Bummer.

## Bites and Stings

### Insect Bites

Whatever creature gets your kid, realize that most children will do just fine and have nothing other than a red, swollen, itchy bite for a while. Ninety-nine percent of the time it honestly doesn't matter what it was that bit your kid. And every kid will react differently. Some children can be attacked by a swarm of mosquitoes and walk away unscathed while others will develop really impressive swelling from just one little bite. Some children are severely allergic to bee stings and can develop difficulty breathing within a matter of minutes while others may just have a bit of soreness at the spot

### 911!

If your little one develops swelling of the lips or tongue, difficulty breathing, becomes unconscious, or otherwise appears to be having a more significant allergic reaction, seek medical attention immediately. Call 911.

where they were stung. As for those kids with nothing more than itchiness and swelling, try a cool compress to alleviate the itching and help with the swelling. An antihistamine by mouth may also be useful.

Certain insects, in particular wasps and bees, may carry the bacteria that cause tetanus, or lockjaw. If your kid has had all his shots, he's probably protected, but if he is older than four and hasn't had his "kindergarten" shots yet, give your doc a call and make sure he doesn't need his booster shots a bit sooner. If in doubt, your pediatrician's office can let you know if your kid is covered.

**Bee Stings.** I sat on a bee once. It hurt. If your kid gets stung, your first clue will probably be a yelp of pain. The dead or dying bee may be there, or all you might see is the stinger. Remove the stinger as fast as possible. It was a long-held belief that stingers should never be pinched because the venom sac might be squeezed, but the newest thinking is that the *speed* of removal is more important than the *method*. A venom sac may continue to release venom for a minute after the sting, so get that thing off your kid as fast as possible, however you need to. Then apply some ice wrapped in a towel to provide pain relief and possibly help to minimize swelling. After that, most kids need only an oral antihistamine and a cool compress, plus a little sympathy.

**911!**

If your kid has a known allergy to bees and gets stung, call your doctor. Use your EpiPen if he develops difficulty breathing, swelling of the lips or tongue, or is unconscious, and then call 911 immediately.

*Spider Bites.* Little Miss Muffet was a histrionic. Don't panic if your kid gets a spider bite. The vast majority of "spider" bites are simply random bug bites and cause nothing more than some pain, redness, and swelling. Black widow spiders can be found worldwide and are large (up to an inch and a half including legs) and have an orange or red hourglass on their bellies. Brown recluse spiders are found in the southern half of the United States and are smaller, dark yellow to brown, and may have a violin-shaped marking on their backs. A black widow spider bite is generally painful and noticed immediately while that of a brown recluse may go unnoticed until symptoms develop, such as a large ulcer of the skin. If you think your kid has been bitten by either of these creatures, give your doctor a call. But for regular old spider bites, treat your kid's symptoms and call your doctor if you think something isn't right.

## Is It Infected?

It can sometimes be difficult to distinguish between an insect bite and an area of skin infection, or cellulitis. Sometimes insect bites can actually become infected. A bug bite is generally going to be itchy. The amount of swelling is not that important because any type of bug bite can cause a significant swelling, such as an eye going totally shut. A bug bite may worsen slightly, with more redness and swelling over the first couple of days, but should then become gradually better. And pus does *not* come out of bug bites, but a little clear fluid might.

## Dog Bites

I don't care how "friendly" a dog is; dogs are animals and will defend or attack if in danger or threatened. Some dogs are naturally more aggressive; pit bulls and rottweilers are vilified as the most aggressive pets around (supported by statistics), although any type of dog can be involved in a serious attack. And it isn't just the kid who is pulling on the dog's tail who gets nipped. It is reported that up to 10 percent of dog bite attacks involve sleeping infants.

If you already own a dog and are bringing a baby into the house, sit down and truly consider whether your dog is going to react in a positive way to the presence of a new arrival. If your dog has a history of aggression of any kind, he and your kid cannot coexist in the same house. Decide which one is more important and get rid of the other. If the kid came first and you are thinking about getting a dog, consider your child's age and personality. If your kid seems frightened of the dog, don't bring it home. Never choose a pet that has a history of aggression, and make sure any dog that joins the family is well socialized and trained in a nonaggressive fashion.

Both parents and dog owners share responsibility for preventing an unfortunate, and possibly fatal, interaction between a child and a dog. Never, ever leave a baby or toddler and a dog unsupervised. Teach your child to avoid unknown dogs. He can have a cookie if he's hungry, but he shouldn't take food out of the dog bowl. Kids should also learn the right way to approach and interact with pets, as well as to remain motionless when approached by a strange or aggressive animal.

## 911!

If your child suffers a dog bite that results in severe bleeding or violence, apply direct pressure to the wounds and call 911.

Unfortunately, the nicest dog and the nicest kid may still come to blows. Even for minor bites, you will probably need to call your doctor. If the wound is bleeding heavily, apply direct pressure for ten to fifteen minutes until the bleeding stops. You can gently clean the wound with soap and plenty of running water. A little bit of bleeding when washing the wound is actually good, because the blood will help wash dirt and bacteria away.

> ## TO STITCH OR NOT TO STITCH
>
> All animal bites carry an increased risk of infection, so the decision to close a wound with stitches is a tough one. We may choose to leave some smaller wounds open even though we would have closed them under other circumstances. It's a matter of balancing the risk of infection with the importance of a good cosmetic outcome. In addition, skin glue should *never* be used to close a bite wound of any kind, because the glue seals in the bacteria and significantly increases the risk of infection.

Call your doctor if a dog bites your kid and she can guide you as to whether the wound requires treatment. Antibiotics are sometimes prescribed for dog bites depending on the type and location of the wound. More important than antibiotics is how vigorously you clean the wound right away, so scrub-a-dub. A simple bandage and some antibiotic ointment may be all that is necessary for very superficial wounds, although some injuries will require a trip to the doctor or the ER. Your doctor can decide if an antibiotic by mouth is necessary.

If your kid has been treated for a dog bite and the wound is becoming more red, swollen, or painful, or if drainage that

is anything other than clear or slightly bloody develops, call
your doctor.

## RABIES

Rabies is a viral illness that is almost uniformly fatal but is,
fortunately, quite rare in the United States and totally prevent-
able with a series of vaccinations after the exposure. The
majority of cases of rabies occur in wild animals, with rac-
coons leading the pack. Skunks, foxes, and coyotes are also
relatively common carriers. Bats are frequent carriers of rabies
and many experts advocate that every potential bat bite
should prompt a physician to initiate the series of injections.
This means that finding a bat in your kid's room is enough to
strongly consider having him vaccinated, even without evidence of a bite. Rabies is very rare in small rodents like rats
and squirrels. A well-appearing bunny is also low risk. However, your kid is probably more likely to come in contact with
a dog or a cat than a wild animal, and both dogs and cats are
rare carriers of rabies. If the animal is a stray or cannot be
located, your child may require vaccination. If you are at all
concerned that your child has been exposed to rabies, call
your pediatrician right away. She will help you decide whether
a vaccination series should be started and where you should
go to initiate treatment.

## Cat Bites

Cats may seem to do nothing but sit around all day and
lick themselves clean but actually they have rather dirty
mouths. Cats also have nice sharp pointy teeth that can puncture more deeply into the skin than those of a dog or another
kid. The teeth of an adult cat occasionally come loose when
chomping into a juicy young child and can become stuck in

the wound. Basically, if your kid suffers a cat bite, you will have to call your doctor. But first clean the wound as vigorously as you can with plenty of running water and soap. Apply pressure to stop the bleeding after you've cleaned the wound and then slap on some antibiotic ointment and a bandage. Letting the wound bleed a bit is actually a good way to remove dirt and bacteria from deep inside the puncture, so go ahead and let the blood run into the sink while you are giving the wound a scrub.

Cat bites are much more likely to become infected than those of a dog. What's more, the bacteria found in a cat's mouth require specific antibiotics. So, if a cat bites your kid, unless it is the most superficial of scratches, your doctor will probably want to prescribe an antibiotic by mouth. Make sure she finishes the entire prescription and let your doctor know immediately if the wound appears more red or painful, develops a pus pocket, or begins to drain.

Of note, kittens (adult cats too, but less likely) often carry a specific bacteria that cause an infection called cat scratch disease. Kids with this infection will develop swelling of lymph nodes, fever, and possibly a rash at the site of a cat scratch, usually within a week or two after contact with an infected cat. Most kids will do just fine, but antibiotic treatment is often necessary. This is another reason to let your pediatrician know about any and all animals with which your little one has contact.

## Human Bites

Cats don't actually have the dirtiest mouths in the animal kingdom. Humans are far filthier. If another child (or adult) bites your kid and the teeth actually break the skin, give the wound a good scrub and call your pediatrician. While many parents immediately freak out about HIV and hepatitis infections, the risk of transmission of these viruses from the saliva is extremely low. The risk of a bacterial infection of the wound is actually much, much higher. However, you can discuss all of these concerns on the phone with your doctor, whom you are dialing right now.

## All the Other Creatures in Your Home

There are some animals that people insist on keeping in their homes and the simple presence of the animal, not just a bite or a scratch, can increase a child's risk of developing a serious infection. The first rule of protecting your kid from one of these infections is never to bring wildlife into the house. *All* pets should come from a breeder or pet store and *never* dragged in from a trip into nature. Wild rabbits, for example, are well-known carriers of certain diseases but these infections are extremely rare in domesticated animals. The biggest problem a pet rabbit will pose for most kids is an allergic reaction. A wild bunny, however, can be a disease-burdened creature you don't want in your home.

Salmonella is an infection that can cause diarrhea in mild cases, or severe illness in those who are very young, old, or immune compromised. While most small rodents are pretty clean when raised in captivity, guinea pigs are surprisingly susceptible to salmonella. Reptiles, such as snakes and lizards, and in particular turtles, are also huge salmonella carriers, meaning they don't get sick but pass the bacteria to anyone with whom they have contact. Salmonella infection is so common in reptiles that you can pretty much assume that any turtle you see will be infected. Make sure your kid washes his hands vigorously and thoroughly after handling his pet turtle, or any animal for that matter.

> **WARNING!**
>
> There have been cases of salmonella in babies who had *no* contact with the reptile in the house, meaning that someone else carried the bacteria from its source to the infant.

All in all, *any* pet can be a potential source of infection to a susceptible person. However, having a pet can be a wonderful and joyful learning experience for a child. Don't let hysteria keep your kid from experiencing the wonders of the animal world. Just make sure that all animals to which your little one is exposed are healthy and domestically reared, and be sure to mention all pets to your doctor or any other health care provider that is tending to your kiddo.

CHAPTER
12

# household poisonings

Well, you knew it would happen eventually. You dutifully installed childproof locks on every door, every cupboard. Shame that your kid is so smart. She waited for that exact moment when your head was turned, when Grandma's purse was open on the floor, and she went for it. Fortunately, most household ingestions are pretty harmless to little kids. And then there are a few items probably lying around your house that can be fatal to a toddler in very small amounts. How are you to know which are which? The answer is extremely difficult. Product labeling is often not terribly helpful. That little pack of silica in your new shoes says "Do not eat" and you would assume this is because it's poisonous and not because you need someone to tell you not to eat things in a shoebox, but it turns out that a little gnawing on that packet isn't going to hurt anyone. (That said, no one should be purposely eating it!) On the other hand, there are lots of things lurking about your home that are surprisingly dangerous.

> **WARNING!**
> A swallowed teaspoon of oil of wintergreen could theoretically kill an entire playgroup. Scary, eh?

## The Culprit

Toddlers are at very high risk for household poisonings because they love to explore and they don't know what is safe and what isn't. What better way to learn about that pretty lipstick in Mommy's makeup bag than to take a big old bite right off the top? Most kids figure out rather quickly that lipstick is a tasteless, oily, mushy, yucky thing, and it is pretty quickly spat right back out onto the carpet. Then again, there are some kids who will eat absolutely anything. My mouth hung open when I saw a seriously ill three-year-old who had actually eaten an *entire* tube of Bengay. Why didn't he stop at one lick? Honestly.

While adolescents are the other group of kids at high risk for poisonings and overdoses, don't forget that a curious and possibly well-meaning toddler can help "feed" the baby. If there is more than one kid in your house, consider them all at risk for an accidental poisoning.

## Preventing Access

There are several types of locks you can buy to keep your curious little one from exploring the drawers and cupboards full of fun and exciting instruments of death. The simplest of locks requires a flip of the finger to release it. Your kid will figure this one out, so it's okay only until he gets past that part of the problem-solving exercise tree. Some locks are actually adhesive, as opposed to screwed into the door. Like a toddler can't figure *that* one out. Some locks fit inside the door and others are visible to your houseguests. Ask for some guidance at the local hardware or baby goods store when choosing a cupboard or drawer lock that is appropriate for the style of the unit. But remember: Your kid will figure it out. This is not a fail-safe or permanent method of keeping him out of harm's way. Respect his ability to work around such small obstacles to fun and keep an eye on him.

Door locks, knob covers, and lever locks are other quick and simple ways to prevent kids from going places they shouldn't. An adult should be able to easily open the door and it must be tough enough to withstand an angry and determined toddler without breaking. That said, most preschoolers can figure them out pretty quickly, and a door lock should *never* substitute for good supervision or be considered a definitive barrier to a swimming pool, a medicine chest, or a knife block. For a good laugh, go read some of the product reviews on Amazon. One parent actually suggested that one supposedly childproof lock be marketed toward the elderly as a device to make opening knobs even easier!

## At the Scene of the Crime

If your child has gotten into something that he shouldn't have, pick him up and remove him from the situation. If he has powder residue on him, brush it off; if it is liquid, wash it off. Many household products, such as rubbing alcohol, can be absorbed through the skin in toxic amounts.

### 911!

If your kid has ingested or been exposed to something such as a medication or chemical and he appears groggy, pale, is having trouble breathing, or you have any other concerns that he is not well, stop reading here and call 911.

Now, assuming that little Billy (goat) is his usual active, happy, destructive self, try to get a handle on the situation. Number one, do you know exactly what he has gotten into? Sometimes this is very easy. For example, you know you left out one bottle of medicine and you know that it was full and you know that everything else is locked away. When you look around, is it *only* the soap bottle that is open? If he got into Grandma's bag, was it *one* container of pills or was it her daily pill sorter that contained five different medicines? It is very important for us to know *what* a child has ingested and this means including all possible household agents or medications in the vicinity. Even if you think the chance is remote, consider it a possibility unless you are absolutely sure that you know exactly what he has taken. Many parents feel so horrendously guilty when they realize their child may have ingested a potentially harmful substance that they will, often subconsciously, try to minimize the situation. You only left him for a minute so he didn't have time to take anything else. He would never, ever do this so it must just be the one item. You were *right there* and pulled a pill out of his mouth, so he definitely didn't have time to swallow one. This is a natural protective response, keeping a parent from feeling the full weight of guilt for what may have happened. Please know, however, that you are *not* alone. Kids do this all the time. It doesn't mean you are bad or neglectful parents. That said, we *do* need to know about anything and everything that he might have taken.

Once you have figured out what he has ingested, are you able to tell how much? If you know how much was in the container before you found him, great. Many times, however, it can be difficult to know how many pills or how much

EMERGENCY!

What if you can't identify a pill or other substance? Call the Poison Center, at 1-800-222-1222. Medications can be identified by codes stamped onto the side of most pills. Other medications are readily identifiable by their size, shape, or color. The fantastic folks answering the phone have access to a specialized computer system that allows a quick and accurate identification of legal medications. If you aren't sure whether there is anything harmful in that thirty-year-old bottle of hair tonic you've been keeping "just in case," they are going to be able to help you with this too. Just have the bottle next to you, ready to describe the size, color, and labeling of the product.

liquid a child has taken. Most toddlers aren't particularly adept at drinking neatly, and most are found with the offending substance all over their faces and shirts. Unfortunately, no matter how much seems to have spilled, we can't accurately measure this amount. Whenever a child is being seen for a suspected ingestion, we have to assume the *largest possible* amount that he could have taken. This is simply for his safety.

At this point, if your child is still well appearing and you know both *what* and *how much* he has probably swallowed, it is time to call your pediatrician or the Poison Center. What is the phone number for your local Poison Center? Nationwide, it's 1-800-222-1222. Where should you put it? Tape it to the phone. No matter what your child has gotten into, no matter what time it is, call this number. Trained professionals who can give you information about every type of poisoning or exposure including bites and stings work at Poison Centers. Once the substance has been identified, the staff can advise you on what to do next. Can you stay home or should you go to the ER? What should you watch for over the next few hours? The Poison Center will often call a family a few hours later to check up and make sure everyone is still okay. Even if you think you know the answer, please double-check. Poison Centers provide an invaluable service, free of charge to you. Both your pediatrician and the Poison Center should be notified immediately of any possible or suspected ingestion in a child.

## TAPE IT TO YOUR PHONE: 1-800-222-1222

Your local Poison Center is reachable twenty-four hours a day by a national toll-free number. This number should be on, or right next to, every phone in your house.

If your doctor or local Poison Center feels that your child may have taken a potentially harmful substance, do *not* panic. Once you arrive at the ER, you should be seen urgently. We have many different ways of protecting patients from the ill effects of being poisoned, although the "stomach pumping" of yesteryear isn't performed all that often. Rather, we have special medications that can absorb many drugs from the stomach and intestines, as well as very specific antidotes for certain medications or poisons. You're heading to the right place, so get there as quickly and *safely* as possible.

### What Is Harmless and What Isn't?

It is not possible to provide a detailed list of all the household products that are generally harmless when ingested in small amounts. Nor would I want to. Many products look alike or have similar-sounding ingredients when they are entirely different and may be extremely toxic. Therefore, no matter what, don't assume a product is harmless and always double-check all information with your pediatrician or Poison Center. On the other hand, there are a surprising number of household items and medications that are extremely dangerous to children, yet will really surprise you. We'll go over a few, but (how many times can I say it?) call your pediatrician or local Poison Center.

## In the Bathroom

Fortunately, most of the stuff that is under the bathroom sink (excluding cleaning supplies) and on your makeup table is nontoxic when eaten in small amounts. Most soaps, shaving creams, shampoos, and bubble baths are okay when swallowed, although your child will probably have some fantastic diarrhea. Your cosmetics, including lipsticks, deodorants, and lotions, are also generally safe. Small amounts of perfume or cologne are generally okay, although they may contain alcohol, which can be quite dangerous for little kids. Some mouthwashes may also be high in alcohol and should be kept up and away from curious tots.

Of course, not everything in there is safe. Rubbing alcohol (isopropyl), even when absorbed through skin, can cause intoxication identical to drinking alcohol (ethanol) but can also cause heart failure and death. Then there is a certain class of molecule called hydrocarbons that are found in industrial chemicals, gasoline, and household products. Hydrocarbons are particularly nasty because if any of the material enters the lung, it can destroy the lung lubricant that allows us to breathe comfortably. A child who has swallowed a substance containing a hydrocarbon may look great at first, but can gradually develop a worsening cough, trouble breathing, or a decrease in the body's oxygen levels. In severe cases, children need to be put on a breathing machine and tragically some children have died. *Of course* you've got some hydrocarbon-containing products in your bathroom. Fortunately, they are probably not the most dangerous forms of these molecules, but still can be quite harmful if accidentally inhaled or ingested in large amounts. Baby oil, suntan oil, and mineral oil are probably in your cupboard right now, so put down the book and go move them to a safe and secure place.

## In the Medicine Cabinet

If he's gotten into the medicine cabinet, which is probably the most dangerous place in the house, there are some medications that are completely safe and others that can be fatal to a toddler in one dose. Remember that childproof caps are not foolproof! Many kids can figure them out without too much difficulty. And why shouldn't they try? Antibiotics taste great! No wonder he just drank a ten-day supply. Check with your doctor, but it's most likely that all you'll need is a new prescription. He doesn't get out of the other nine days just by drinking the bottle today. And you will definitely want to refill your birth control pills when he's finished eating the pack. Most oral contraceptives will cause vomiting in an overdose but are unlikely to be harmful to your little Bubby.

Every household with kids has a bottle of either acetaminophen (such as Tylenol) or ibuprofen (such as Advil or Motrin). Both medications are extremely safe and effective when taken in appropriate dosages. What if he drinks the whole bottle? An entire bottle of ibuprofen might cause some stomach upset, or rarely bleeding or kidney problems. However, most kids who have overdosed on a moderate amount of ibuprofen do very well and do not require emergency treatment. Acetaminophen, on the other hand, can be quite toxic when taken in overdose. Medication to block the effects of acetaminophen on the liver may need to be started right away, depending on the suspected amount taken, and laboratory testing will be performed to measure the amount of acetaminophen in the body. If the detected amount is high enough, the medication will continue until all the acetaminophen has been cleared from the body, which usually can take two to three days. Acetaminophen is a really great, safe medication to have in your armory, but remember to lock it up. Just because it is made for children doesn't necessarily mean it is safe in overdoses!

EMERGENCY!

A child who may have ingested a "toxic" amount of acetaminophen (as calculated by your doctor on a special chart, or nomogram) will need emergency evaluation. Call your Poison Center (1-800-222-1222) or your pediatrician right away.

Unfortunately, most other medications may be quite harmful, whether he takes too many doses of his own medicine or just one tablet of yours. Any medications that are for treating heart or blood pressure problems can be deadly to a small child. Same for medications used to treat diabetes. Some antidepressants are relatively safe while others, particularly in the *tricyclic* family, can be deadly. Iron is a common

## BEWARE OF COMBO DRUGS

Many products containing ibuprofen or acetaminophen may contain other drugs, such as cough and cold preparations. These other medications can be toxic in their own right, so be sure to list *every* ingredient when speaking to your pediatrician or Poison Center about a possible or suspected ingestion by your wee pup.

and potentially fatal ingestion in children, who may find an adult preparation of iron pills that look disturbingly like candy.

Any medication or other product containing aspirin or an aspirin-related substance can cause aspirin poisoning in a small child. Adult Pepto-Bismol is an example of a common medication that contains an aspirinlike medication although it is generally not highly toxic when taken in a small amount. (However, Pepto-Bismol can actually be *seen* on an X-ray, so fess up if you gave him some!) Conversely, oil of wintergreen, used as a muscle ache or headache treatment, contains an extremely concentrated form of aspirin and a tiny sip could be deadly to a child.

Medications that are meant to relax you, such as muscle relaxants or sedatives (like Valium), might make a child so

## WARNING!

Some medications that can be particularly dangerous for little kids in very small doses include heart and blood pressure medicines, diabetes pills, tricyclic antidepressants, "relaxing" medicines (such as Valium), and pain medications (pill, gel, or cream).

"relaxed" that he forgets to breathe. Pain medications containing narcotics, such as codeine or morphine, might also cause such profound "relaxation" that they could be fatal to a little one. Interestingly, many drugs contain these compounds without your realizing what exactly is in there. Loperamide, a drug found in some anti-diarrheal medications, can be fatal to a toddler if taken in adult doses. Another group of "pain" medicine includes the numbing medicines for mouth sores and creams or salves for muscle pain. Teething gels designed for babies are very safe when used as directed, but the active ingredient (benzocaine) can be extremely dangerous and potentially could be fatal to a small child if taken in the wrong dose. Certain preparations of "pain" medications in a gel or cream, such as muscle rubs, can lead to uncontrollable seizures or, in rare cases, death, even if ingested in small amounts.

This is in no way an exhaustive list of medications that could be harmful to your child, but is just meant to highlight a few of the more common, and fatal, medications you may have at home. When it comes to medicines, be they in your purse, at Grandma's house, or in your bathroom cupboard, take no chances. Lock them up! And if he picks the lock, call your pediatrician or Poison Center immediately.

## In the Kitchen

It's not just the knives on the kitchen counter that can harm a child. There's plenty of danger lurking in your cupboards and under the sink! I don't have to tell you to lock up the wine, beer, and liquor. Not only is it inappropriate to laugh at a drunk two-year-old, but alcohol ingestion in kids should be treated very seriously. Alcohol can cause a severe drop in blood sugar, which can be very dangerous for an active little kid who doesn't have the massive sugar stores in her muscles and liver that you and I keep. Kids move all the time, so they burn through their energy stores very quickly and have very little reserve. A toddler will not only fail to appreciate a nice glass of wine, but might find himself needing an IV of sugar water until the alcohol has been metabolized. A classic scenario in the ER is the drunk kid on New Year's Day. Wee Jasper's parents had a party, half-drunk cups were left lying around, he woke up before his folks, went into the living room, and started his own little party. It doesn't take much alcohol to intoxicate a toddler!

### WARNING!
It's not just your whiskey that has alcohol, by the way. Vanilla extract can have a higher alcohol concentration than many liqueurs!

Most of us keep our household cleaning supplies in the kitchen under the sink. If your kid goes exploring under there, most soap products are safe, as are some detergents. However, other soaplike cleaning products may cause burning of the mouth and esophagus that can be quite severe. On the other hand, household bleach is actually quite dilute and a small swig is harmless, although ingesting larger volumes or industrial-strength products can be dangerous. Remember the hydrocarbons? Furniture polish and oils may contain hydrocarbons, so be sure to keep these products away from children. Finally, lamp oil looks pretty and smells nice but is very dangerous. Either fill your lamps with water and food coloring, or put them away until your child moves out.

**WARNING!**

Toilet bowl and drain cleaners may be very damaging if taken in even a small sip, as can furniture polish and other cleaning "oils." Decorative lamp oils are very pretty and look quite cool but are also deadly if ingested.

If you find that your child has gotten into any of your general cleaning products, whether he drank something or poured it all over himself, get him cleaned up quickly and call your doctor or Poison Center, at 1-800-222-1222.

## In the Family Room

Fortunately, the "family room" is a pretty safe place for a kid. Paste, glue, crayons, ballpoint pens, paper, and pretty much everything else he can find in his sister's backpack is perfectly safe when eaten in small amounts. Your biggest problem when he's found chewing on a permanent marker is explaining his green lips and tongue for the next few days. However, some of these products may come from unconventional sources (remember that vacation in Mexico?) or have hidden ingredients, so don't panic, but do give your pediatrician a call if he's eaten his way through the arts and crafts desk.

**EMERGENCY!**

Disc batteries are commonly ingested or stuck into noses or ears and can be very dangerous if left unrecognized. For more information on which foreign bodies are dangerous and which aren't, check out Chapter 5 and the discussion on stuff in your kid's nose.

And if he's glued his arm to something, no worries. While most regular glues and pastes are okay to taste in small amounts, what is a parent to do when her kid gets into the really good stuff, like Super Glue? I once took a phone call from a chap at another hospital who was tending to a two-year-old who had poured the stuff all over his front and literally glued his pants on. After I finished wiping my tears of laughter, I called my friendly Poison Center to ask for some advice, and when they were done laughing, we all decided that the best thing to do would be to pour salad oil all over his pants and stick him in the tub. Honestly, superpowerful glues are very useful medically—we can use them to repair cuts and hold together wounds. It won't actually *hurt* your child if he glues his eye shut, or his shirt is stuck to his arm. With time, the glue will begin to flake away and the old skin will begin to slough off and things will separate. If you can't wait that long, salad oil or petroleum jelly might break down the glue more quickly, as will keeping the area wet. A smudge of petroleum jelly on the eyelid can be covered with a bandage if he's smearing it around. Don't just freak out and pull the stuck pieces apart, because you will probably rip his skin and make him cry. Just keep the area as wet and oily as you can and keep calm. Oh, and call your pediatrician or Poison Center both to ensure that the particular glue formulation is safe *and* to give everyone else a good chuckle.

As I've said, the family room is a pretty safe place when it comes to household poisonings. He can even eat the fish food. So let's move on.

## In the Garage

Kids should not be playing in the garage unattended. Period. There are too many dangers lurking in every corner.

Not to mention his Christmas presents. In one corner sits the antifreeze, which tastes yummy and can be fatal, and in the other corner sits a can of spare gasoline, a deadly hydrocarbon. On the tool bench is a container of paint remover, which contains a dangerous type of alcohol, and a can of turpentine, another hydrocarbon. Next to your camping equipment are a container of kerosene and a can of lighter fluid (hydrocarbons). Stove fuels, such as Sterno, contain a deadly alcohol. Finally, please tell me that there are no unmarked mystery fluids lying around. Many household accidents result from children getting into something brought home from a parent's workplace. To sum it up, the garage is a pretty difficult place to childproof, so keep the door locked.

In summary, kids are curious and want to learn about everything. Unfortunately, they do this often with their mouths. If your kid has gone "exploring," do *not* panic, remove him from the situation, and immediately call your pediatrician or Poison Center, at 1-800-222-1222. Chances are that there is nothing to be done, but occasionally a child will need emergent evaluation and treatment, and that decision is best left to the professionals.

# mama, owie!

## Minor Bumps, Bruises, Burns, and Wounds

Fortunately, most trauma to little kids is minor. That is good because it is really common. Kids fall down, they cut themselves, they touch hot glowing things. They seem to have a limited comprehension of cause and effect. While broken bones and major injuries are covered in Chapter 14, the visible consequences of reckless juvenile behavior can be found in this chapter, along with a few tips on what to expect from your doctor or emergency room should this injury require treatment.

### Simple Wounds

#### Bumps and Bruises

Underneath our skin is a whole world of fat cells and blood vessels, sweat glands, fibrous things like collagen, and other cells and structures of the body. These all combine to support and nourish our skin, help control our body temperature, and keep us waterproof. Just as with anyplace in the body, however, injury to the skin can not only cause breakage of blood vessels, but also result in a whole host of "inflammatory responders" (like blood cells) flocking to the injured area in an attempt to set things right again. This means that even a little bump or bonk can cause impressive bruising and swelling. Areas where the skin is looser, such as around the eyes, will become more bruised and swollen appearing than other areas where the skin is more taut, because there is simply more room for the blood and fluid to congregate. Similarly, areas that have a richer blood supply, such as the face and head, can also develop pretty impressive bruising and swelling in response to injury.

There are very few bumps and bruises that require any form of treatment. With a few exceptions, symptomatic treatment of the pain or discomfort is all that is needed. An age- and weight-appropriate dose of a pain medicine such as acetaminophen or ibuprofen will be helpful. Ibuprofen has the added benefit of being an "anti-inflammatory," meaning that it may help not only with the pain, but also with the swelling.

### Ice

Cold packs or ice may help reduce the flow of blood to an injured area, thereby possibly decreasing the amount of swelling. You can buy a commercial cold pack, use the chill-pack that came with your caviar order last week, or stick some ice cubes in a plastic baggie. Frozen vegetables, like peas, also work really well. Popsicles are great for mouth injuries. It doesn't really matter what form of cold you use. What matters is that ice and other very cold things should *never* be held in direct contact with the skin, because it could indeed burn the skin. Make sure there is something between the skin and the cold pack, such as a towel, and don't leave the pack on for more than twenty minutes at a time.

If your kid has taken a good whack to the head, the same rules about head injuries apply and you don't necessarily have to call your doctor only to report swelling or bruising. However, injury and significant bruising to the upper part of the ear could damage the soft bone, or cartilage, and may require evaluation by a specialist. Bruising or swelling of the neck could, rarely, make it difficult to breathe if the swelling is very large. Finally, swelling that cuts off blood supply to the fingers or toes could cause serious injury. This condition is called compartment syndrome, and occurs when blood and bodily fluids fill up the spaces between the muscles in the arm or leg so tightly that blood in the veins and arteries can't get through. This is extremely unlikely to happen in the absence of a broken bone, but if your kid has his arm rolled over by his sister's bike and develops significant bruising and swelling of the arm (usually all the way around), check to make sure that his little fingers can wiggle, are nice and warm and pink, and it doesn't hurt him when you straighten them. As always, if you are ever in doubt as to whether a bruise or an area of swelling needs tending to, call your pediatrician.

## Abrasions and Lacerations

All children will, at some point, either cut or scrape themselves up. Be it with a knife, broken glass, an unforeseen meeting with the pavement, or even an innocent-looking piece of paper, your kid will injure himself at some point in his existence. You can't cover him in bubble wrap. If the cut is bleeding very heavily, apply direct pressure to control the bleeding and seek medical attention. Remember that cuts to the head and face will bleed a lot, since we have such a fabulous blood supply above the neck. So, by "bleeding very heavily," I mean spurting blood, puddles of blood, blood spraying the walls. That kind of bleeding deserves a phone call to 911. All other bleeding deserves a few minutes of firm pressure over the wound and then you can take a peek. But give it a good couple of minutes. Sneak a look too soon and you will cause yourself unnecessary worry.

If little Rocky comes strolling in from the playground covered with blood, the first question you should ask yourself is "Where is the bleeding coming from?" If the answer is "From my kid," then you must ask yourself whether the injury is going to require medical treatment. There are a couple of factors that help us decide whether a child is going to require stitches, or sutures. The first is whether there is anything to sew back together. Think about splitting your pants. You can sew the seam back together, right? But what about the knees of your jeans, where the material has worn away and now there is a hole. You couldn't sew the two sides of that together, could you? Sometimes a cut will look like its edges are very far apart but the skin will actually come together very nicely. However, if the injury actually resulted in more of a *scraping* away of the skin, then there won't be anything to suture.

A scraping of the skin is called an abrasion and usually requires only a good cleaning and bandaging. Since he probably scraped himself up outside, in the dirt and rocks, you might need to pop him into the tub for a good soak to get all the bits of grime and grit out of the wound. After you have cleaned him up, you can apply a little antibiotic ointment (if it's handy) and a bandage. For the pain, try some acetaminophen or ibuprofen and maybe a cold pack or some ice (but *never* directly to the skin!). Very rarely will an abrasion be so large and deep that it actually will require skin grafting, but

## SUNSCREEN

New skin has to grow in and heal any cut or scrape, no matter how tiny. It can take a good six months before a wound is fully healed. Now, would you put your naked newborn out on a beach towel in Arizona? No. Keep new skin protected from the sun by covering it with clothing or a hat, keeping it in the shade, or by using sunscreen until the area has completely healed. As skin heals, scar tissue will form and is much more susceptible to sun exposure, turning darker more quickly than the old skin.

this would happen only with severe injuries and occur later, not on an emergent basis.

For cuts, or lacerations, we will consider both the size and depth of the cut as well as how far apart the edges are. A very short cut that has the edges already stuck back together probably isn't going to benefit from a stitch, although if it is continuing to open and bleed, then it may need closing. A longer cut that is very shallow might also not need much more than a couple of strips of bandage to keep the edges together while it heals. Kids heal really fast, especially on their head and face, and most small cuts will be pretty well stuck together within three to five days. If you aren't sure whether his injury is going to require stitches, call your doctor. The faster we can repair a cut, the less likely that it will get infected or have problems healing. In fact, we have rules about how long after an injury a cut should be repaired, so don't delay treatment.

Whether your kid's injury needs treatment or not, any break in the skin can put a person at risk for tetanus, a disease that causes uncontrollable muscle spasms and other nasty symptoms. Tetanus used to be known as lockjaw, because patients would develop spasms of the jaw muscles. In developing countries, tetanus is not uncommon and children often die if infected. In the United States, tetanus is quite rare but does occur, usually in children who were not immunized or elderly folk who haven't had a booster shot in years. If your kid has cut himself in any way, double-check with your doctor about his tetanus immunity. If he's had his shots at the correct times, he's probably okay, although he will need a booster shot between four and six years old. If he hasn't had his "kindergarten shots" yet and he's about that age, he might need to get his shots bumped up. But don't worry about rushing to the ER in the middle of the night or on a weekend; it's okay to wait until your pediatrician's office is open Monday morning.

### WOUND INFECTIONS

Any cut or scrape has the potential to become infected. Increasing pain, swelling, pus, red streaks, or redness around the wound demands a call to your doctor.

## Putting Humpty Back Together

If you are pretty sure that your kid is going to need his wound repaired, or if your doctor has seen the injury and is sending you to the hospital, it is a good idea to try to prepare your child. The first thing he is going to ask is "Will it hurt?" The correct answer here is, "Gosh, I hope not, but we'll have to ask the doctor about how she's going to make it as painless as possible." The wrong answers are "Yes" or "No." You should expect that your kid will receive some type of pain medication, either by mouth or directly to the wound. However, sometimes the administration of pain medicine can be slightly painful. What is more, even with a very good local anesthetic, a person will feel pressure and pulling. It is always a good idea to be honest with a child and tell him that he might feel something but all the bad pain should be gone. Or you can feign total ignorance and let us do the talking. It's a good idea to bring a book or other distracting toys or games with you to keep your kid occupied both before and during treatment.

Depending on what the practice is at your local emergency room, and depending on where the wound is, a numbing jelly might be applied about a half hour before any cleaning or sutures. The medicine is cold and can sting for just a minute, but then works wonderfully to numb the top layers of skin.

Sometimes the numbing jelly isn't available. Other times it can't be applied because of the location of the injury due to its tendency to restrict local blood flow. Some cuts are so deep that the jelly might not have numbed the area adequately and additional medication will be injected directly into the injury. When any type of fluid is injected into the skin, the stretching and pressure can cause some pain, which is worsened by the stinging nature of most local anesthetics. So, it is normal for a kid to give a yelp at this point, but the pain is gone within seconds.

Finally, the wound will be cleaned and repaired. There are several options for wound repair, including traditional stitches, special skin glue, or a medical staple gun (not the one in your desk or out in the garage!). Which of these we choose to use depends on the age of the kid, the location and size of the wound, the mechanism of injury, and a host of other factors. Regardless of the way in which the wound is repaired, the

## SUPERGLUE

Most parents have heard about the fabulous skin glue that can be used to close many cuts. The glue is faster to apply, doesn't hurt, and falls away on its own, obviating the need for suture removal. However, before you get all excited, you should know that wounds that are larger or deeper will probably require traditional stitches, as well as those on areas of "tension," such as over knuckles, knees, or other areas that bend and move. Spots that are very wet, such as in and around the mouth, are also not good locations for skin glue. The glue is inappropriate for cuts with a higher risk of infection, such as human or animal bites.

nurse or doctor should give you follow-up care instructions and let you know if you'll need to return to the ER or your doctor's office for a wound check or to have stitches or staples removed.

If a wound is particularly complicated or in an area of extreme cosmetic importance, some ER doctors will decide to call a plastic surgeon for assistance with the repair. It is okay to ask if your child should have his wound repaired by a surgeon specializing in cosmetic wound repair, but do know that most cuts on kids are going to heal extremely well with very little scarring and most doctors working in an emergency room are quite adept at wound repair. Also, you should know that *all* cuts and wounds scar to some extent, regardless of who performs the repair. In some centers there are actually designated physician assistants or technicians who do nothing but sew little kids back together and are fantastic. I would absolutely let these guys sew up my face. Finally, in some academic hospitals, the "plastic surgeon" who responds to the call is in reality a junior doctor-in-training and may have less experience than the ER staff when it comes to repairing little kids' wounds.

# Burns

## Classifying Burns

A burn is an injury to the skin that can be classified by the depth to which it penetrates. A superficial burn, including only the top layers of skin, is called a first-degree burn, and results in redness and pain but no blistering of the skin, such as a mild sunburn. A second-degree burn causes injury to the deeper skin layers and can cause intense pain, redness, and blistering. Burns that go deeper than the deep layers of the skin may cause injury to the underlying nerves, muscle, or bone. These injuries are sometimes referred to as third- and fourth-degree burns. Any burn deeper than a second-degree burn will be more serious and may have a white or burned appearance. These deeper burns are often painless, since the nerves under the skin have been burned away.

## EMERGENCY!

Any burn deeper than a second-degree burn will absolutely require medical attention and often surgery and skin grafting to replace the permanently injured skin.

A burn can occur from exposure to heat or cold, electrical forces, or exposure to certain chemicals. The extremity of the temperature and the time of exposure of the skin will determine how deep the injury goes. All burns, be they from heat, cold, electrical shocks, or the sun, are diagnosed and treated in basically the same way.

*Thermal Burns.* Thermal burns happen when something very hot comes in contact with the skin long enough to cause a burn. Hot water, boiling soup, piping hot pizza, and glowing BBQ coals are all potential causes of a thermal burn.

By setting your water heater to a maximum temperature of 120°F, you can significantly increase the amount of time it takes to cause a severe hot water burn. This is plenty warm enough for you to take a nice long shower and still a simple and fantastically effective means of protecting your offspring. Remember that the bathtub isn't the only source of potentially scalding liquid at home. Keep all handles on the stove turned inward, away from little hands. Same goes for your coffee cup on the table. An adult holding a hot pan of grease can easily trip over a tottering child, so keep the mobile, yet safety unaware, out of the way while you are cooking. A playpen or bouncy chair is good for this purpose. And don't even think that you can balance a squirming child in one hand and a cup of hot tea in the other. Recipe for disaster.

> ### EMERGENCY!
> Smoke inhalation can occur in kids exposed to fire, so if the injury is the result of something burning, like your house, don't be completely distracted by his injuries. Coughing or breathing hard, ashes and soot around the mouth or nose, or a hoarse voice are all signs that a child's airways and lungs may have been injured. Call your doctor or 911.

*Sunburn.* The guilt from letting your kid cook all day on the beach will stick with you for a while. Sunburns in childhood are associated with an increased risk of skin cancer in adults. The American Academy of Pediatrics recommends that everyone cover up and stay in the shade during hours of peak sun intensity. Right. Okay. At the very least, kids should be covered in sunscreen with an SPF of *at least* 15, applied thirty minutes before going outside and reapplied every two hours or after sweating or swimming. We all should be wearing a floppy hat, sunglasses, and long, lightweight clothing. Babies under six months *can* have small amounts of sunscreen applied to the areas that you can't cover with clothing, such as faces and backs of hands. Try to remember that the younger the kid, the greater the risk of heat-related injury and sunburn, so babies should be parked in the shade and kept cool yet covered.

If your child has turned into a lobster while looking for one, get him out of the sun as soon as you can. Cool the skin down, either with a cold damp cloth or a cool bath or shower (a forceful spray will sting!). A cool drink and quiet rest will make him feel better and an age-appropriate dose of ibuprofen will help with the pain and inflammation of his skin. Periodic application of cool compresses will also make him more comfortable.

The vast majority of sunburns can be managed at home and cause only a few days of suffering. However, sunburns can be quite severe, so if the burned area is very large and blistered, your doctor may want to see your kid the following day. The younger the baby, the more worrisome overexposure to the sun becomes. Babies have a lot more skin in relation to the size of their bodies, so a burn can be more severe, and they don't sweat effectively, making them more likely to overheat. A sunburn in a younger infant or any burn that is more than mild should probably be brought to your doctor's attention. The combination of having been overheated all day, a large burn, and feeling too miserable to drink properly can put any child at risk for developing dehydration, so be sure to encourage plenty of liquids. If you are worried that your little one is suffering from a sunburn that is beyond what you feel comfortable managing, or you are worried that he may be suffering from heat exhaustion or heat stroke, don't hesitate to call your doctor.

## HEAT STROKE AND EXHAUSTION

Heat-related illnesses range from just a leg cramp to more serious conditions such as heat exhaustion and finally heat stroke, which can be tragically fatal. If your kid has been exposed to hot conditions, such as playing rough on the beach or sitting in a parked car, and develops fever, headache, vomiting, extreme fatigue or lethargy, or confusion, call your doctor right away.

*Cold Burns.* I once took care of a really dumb kid who got into a pain contest with some of his buddies. They each poured salt onto their hands, then held an ice cube on the skin. The last one to stand the pain won. Well, what he won was a full-thickness burn to the back of his hand that required skin grafting. Skin injury from cold exposure can be mild and temporary (called chilblain), which is basically what happens when you play outside in the snow and come inside with burning cheeks. Longer or more severe exposure can result in injury to deeper layers of the skin and these injuries are commonly called frostnip or frostbite. Burns from exposure to ice or extreme temperatures can be just as severe as those due to any other cause. For all forms of cold injury, the area needs to be rewarmed, but *not* until you can be sure that the skin won't refreeze. Unless you are stuck in an avalanche, this probably doesn't pertain, but I thought I should mention it.

Your doctor should definitely hear about any injury from exposure to cold conditions or contact with a frozen item that is more severe than a superficial redness that goes away simply by coming inside and covering up. Ice crystals within the skin cells can cause significant injury and your child should probably be checked out.

*Chemical Burns.* Exposure to chemicals that are either very acidic or very alkaline, such as lime or wet cement, can cause injury to the skin. Even a really potent clove of garlic could burn little Tony's hand if left in contact with his delicate skin for too long. Regardless of what the offending agent is, the first-line management of a burn due to contact with a chemical is to wash the skin and remove any trace of the substance. Rinse with water for ten to fifteen minutes or longer while you are phoning your pediatrician or local Poison Center, at 1-800-222-1222. Depending on what the chemical is and how large the injury, your little one may need urgent evaluation.

## Simple Burn Management

Regardless of the mechanism of the burn, the first thing you should do is to separate the burned part from whatever is burning it. Specific immediate care depends on the type of burn.

## ⑨ | | !

If your kid is unconscious or having trouble breathing, has a burn that is covering a very large part of his body or his hands, feet, face, or genitals, call your doctor or 911.

**WARNING!**

Do *not* put butter, lard, Crisco, oil, or any of the other "home" remedies on a burn. They not only will *not* help, but can make the situation much worse.

For superficial, or first-degree, burns, cool the area as quickly as you can. Running cold water or cold wet towels are fine. This not only will stop the area from burning any further but will help immensely with the pain. You can then apply a little antibiotic ointment, which will be soothing and moisturizing. Pain control with acetaminophen or ibuprofen would be appropriate, and a good bandage will help to protect the area. A burn that has gone deeper and created a blister, if it is still relatively minor, can be treated with a simple bandage. Don't pop the blister, although if the skin has broken open, you can very gently remove any dead bits, as long as it doesn't cause too much pain. Any burn that is more severe than a few superficial blisters will require evaluation by your doctor and possibly referral to a specialist. If you are at all in doubt, call your pediatrician.

**ANTIBIOTICS?**

Even though our biggest concern with healing wounds is the development of an infection, burns should not be treated with preventative antibiotics, with the exception of an antibiotic ointment. Antibiotics by mouth should be given *only* to kids who have signs of an infection. Preemptive antibiotic treatment won't prevent an infection but will make any infection that develops more difficult to treat.

If you've managed to deal with a minor burn on your own, be sure to change the bandage daily and watch for signs of infection such as worsening redness (especially of the skin *around* the burn), green or yellow drainage, or worse pain. Some pinkness at the edges and within the burn is normal and is a sign of healthy new skin growing. However, deeper pink or red, especially if more tender or warm, may signify infection. If any of these signs occur, call your doctor promptly.

### GREEN GOOP

If your kid has been seen for a burn, he may have been given a special burn cream called silver sulfadiazine (or Silvadene). Silvadene is great for helping more significant burns heal, but beware! The compound contains silver, which can actually impart a shiny, silvery look to the skin. What's more, as the wound drains and mixes with the cream, it can form a greenish material. Don't be fooled into thinking this is an infection if the wound is otherwise healing nicely, there is no worsening pain or redness, and your child is otherwise well.

# major trauma and accident prevention

No matter how hard you work to protect your child, she will find a way to injure herself. Broken bones, split-open chins, and a few good bumps to the head are rites of passage. Unfortunately, trauma can sometimes be serious and even threaten a child's survival. In fact, injuries are the number one cause of death in the United States for kids under four. But even in cases of potentially life-threatening injury, many children will prove surprisingly resilient. Take a breath. We'll talk about a few of the extremely frightening situations in which a child may find himself and what you need to know in the moment. More important, I'll tell you what, if any, steps you might have taken to prevent harm in the first place.

## Falls

Kids are pretty rubbery. I once saw a kid who fell out of the second-story window and then crawled (crying) around to

> **911!**
> If you fear that your child has suffered a major injury, is unconscious, is bleeding profusely, is not breathing, or is having trouble breathing, call 911 immediately.

## How Far They Fall

Those of us who work with pediatric emergencies have a rule: Under three months, over three feet. A doctor should see all babies younger than twelve weeks who fall from an estimated height of over a yard.

knock on the front door. Not every kid is so lucky. Whether from a tree, a piece of playground equipment, or the top of your refrigerator, little kids will fall down. The good news is that a small child's body is made to fall. They are short, so they don't have far to go until they hit the ground, plus they are covered in all kinds of padding. Heck, they even come with a set of teeth they can knock out! However, babies and kids have heads that are disproportionately large compared to the rest of their bodies, meaning they will usually tumble downward headfirst. Like the anticat.

Even though most falls are quite innocent, falling from a significant height might cause severe, even life-threatening, injury in children. But if she gets up on her own and seems to be moving all her pieces and parts, she's likely fine. If you are at all worried that she may have broken a bone or has injured her head, give your doctor a call (while reading about head injuries and broken bones).

## 911!

If your little one takes a tumble and is unconscious or refusing to move, don't pick her up. Keep her still and calm, and call 911.

## The Stairs

One place kids love to fall is on the staircase. Parents always want to know, "How many steps are dangerous when falling?" The answer is, "It doesn't matter." The first step is the most important. After that one, the number becomes largely irrelevant. Either you hurt yourself or you don't.

If your kid falls down the stairs, the same rules as above apply. If she's not moving or appears seriously injured, call 911. Otherwise, see how she's doing. A happy, laughing kid (once she stops crying) is fine. If in doubt, call your pediatrician.

### BABY GATES

If your house has stairs and you have a baby, you probably have a baby gate. Good. Try to actually *use* it. While a pain to constantly step over, baby gates are a great way to help keep your little one safe. But don't rely solely on the gate to keep your kid from a tumble. If he's old enough to push or pull his booster seat over to the gate, he's old enough to launch himself down the stairs. Never become complacent.

*Preventing Falls.* All windows above ground level and those that can be accessed by a small child should be fitted with a window lock, which should still allow you to open the window enough to air out the little stinker's room, but prevent him from making an escape. Make sure that any window guard or lock is easily operable by an adult, to allow for escape in case of fire or other emergency.

If you have a changing table, your child will fall off it. Maybe not today, maybe not tomorrow, but it will happen. Babies seem to learn to roll the minute they are placed on an elevated surface. Always keep *at least* one hand firmly on

## CORNER BUMPERS

Beware of sharp edges. Get down on all fours and crawl around, looking for corners (such as on a table or fireplace) where a kid could bonk his head. An edge bumper won't keep your kid from falling or hitting his head, but might keep you out of the ER.

your little one while you search for lotion, wipes, and the like. Either that, or change him on the floor.

A rather significant number of injuries happen to babies who use infant walkers. The most common injury is probably the worst: a tumble down the staircase. Newer walkers are supposedly "safer" than previous models, but serious injury still can occur. To add insult to injury, using an infant walker does *not* teach a baby to walk sooner. In fact, it may actually *delay* little JoJo's first steps. Babies need to spend time rolling around on the floor, developing their trunk muscles so they have enough strength to hold themselves erect. If you want to confine your kid to one place while you make dinner (because, let's be honest, there's your motive), consider a stationary activity center without wheels. If you absolutely refuse to listen and are committed to using a walker, at least try to find one that is wider than the doorframe and make sure it has working wheel locks. Older models may have areas that can pinch or catch a bit of baby skin, so check for sharp edges, springs, or other spots that might hurt. Always be present when your child is in the walker and watch out for hot or dangerous objects within her newfound reach, such as a radiator or a box of scissors. Or just listen to the medical consensus and don't use one.

## Automobile Accidents

So you passed the baby a cookie and now you've run down the neighbor's mailbox. I don't need to lecture you on being a safe, defensive driver. Yet, despite your best efforts to keep your infant and child safe while riding in a moving vehicle, sometimes the neighbor's mailbox is just going to jump out of nowhere and smack into your car. So what do you do?

If the collision was minor and everyone was suitably restrained, the chance of an injury that requires medical attention is slim. Even in significant impacts, a properly restrained child who appears well and is moving about is likely fine. A lot of kids will complain of some mild neck pain in the hours to days after a car accident, which is most often muscle tenderness, but these kids will usually feel pretty good and not have any trouble moving their neck at the time of the accident.

### 911!

A kid who is unconscious, blue, bleeding, or having trouble breathing after an automobile collision needs emergency care immediately. A kid who refuses to turn his head or move his neck at the scene of the accident should *not* be moved and EMS should be called.

If you get out of the car and everyone seems fine, albeit startled, it should be up to you and the rescue crews to decide who needs to be seen emergently. A child who has been in a car accident and is complaining of belly pain or has blood in his urine needs to be seen by a doctor, even if several hours later. Any bruising along the path of the seat belt, especially if on the tummy, needs to be checked out. If you are in any doubt, call your pediatrician. Remember that having a correctly installed and age-appropriate car seat is one of the easiest things you can do to keep your kid safe.

## Safety-Restraint Systems

It is pretty rare to see a baby or young child severely injured in a motor vehicle accident if properly restrained in a correctly installed, age- and weight-appropriate child safety seat. This doesn't mean that a car seat is a guarantee that your child will survive a severe automobile collision, but happy, uninjured babies have been found ejected from a car and upside down while still properly strapped into their car seats. The seat belt may have failed, but the infant-restraint system did not. This evidence has convinced me that properly restraining a child can be absolutely lifesaving. The type of car seat you choose is dependent upon the age and weight of your child and the type of vehicle in which you are traveling. Any chosen safety-restraint system should be relatively new and in good condition, have no damaged or missing parts, and have never been part of a recall. Any car seat that has survived a moderate to severe car crash should be considered unsafe and potentially damaged.

### ESSENTIAL INFORMATION

An excellent and very thorough guide to choosing and installing a car seat, as well as safety tips and answers to common questions, can be found on the American Academy of Pediatrics Web site: www.aap.org. Another helpful site belongs to the National Highway Traffic Safety Administration (www.nhtsa.dot.gov), where you can find information on product recalls, locate a car seat fitting station, or learn more about car seat safety and "Ease of Use" ratings.

### Quick Car-Seat Reference

- Infants *always* ride rear-facing until they are at least one year old *and* at least twenty pounds. The longer you can keep him looking where he's already been, the safer he'll be. When he can stick his legs out the bottom of the seat and start pushing up and out with any degree of strength, flip him around.

- Little kids should be in a forward-facing car seat until they can verbalize embarrassment. The longer they stay that way, the safer they are. Minimum age and weight for moving to a booster seat are four years and forty pounds. If your kid outgrows his car seat before he reaches an age of humiliation, he needs to move to a booster.

- Bigger kids need to be in a booster until they are about four feet, nine inches tall and the adult seat belt fits well. For most kids, this means at *least* eight years old.

- Everyone else should wear an adult seat belt, which should absolutely include both a lap and a shoulder harness. The shoulder belt should never go *behind* the kid (or the adult).

- Anyone under the age of thirteen should be in the backseat. Airbags save lives, but can kill those too tiny to handle the force of an expanding bag. If you absolutely must use the front seat, make sure the airbag is disengaged. The explosive power of an airbag could cause your little one far greater injury than the accident itself.

## Bikes and Riding Toys

I cringe when I look back at those family photos, me two years old and happily waving from the carrier seat on the back of my dad's bike, hair blowing in the breeze, Pop's wide-bottomed pant leg flapping wildly around the bike chain. Where was my helmet? Why is my dad wearing those orange checkered pants? The rules on bike (and riding toy) safety have changed dramatically since the ancient days of my childhood, and for the better. Bike helmets save lives. And it's not just the older child who is at risk from bikes and other riding craft. Babies and little kids can find themselves unwilling victims of serious injury.

The rules are pretty simple. All kids, regardless of age, need a helmet when riding on or behind a bicycle. If you choose to use a rear-mounted seat on your bike, the seat should be sturdy, properly attached, have a strong, and child-proof, safety belt, and be equipped with spoke guards to protect little fingers and toes. However, many experts recommend against using a rear-mounted seat for any child, and babies under one year of age definitely shouldn't ride in one. A child trailer is not only a safer alternative, but the drag may help you burn a few extra calories. Any trailer should be specifically designed for kids, be equipped with a safety harness, and be able to accommodate a sleeping kid wearing a helmet without allowing his head to loll off to the side.

Once you've got your kid all tucked into his protective shell, keep the cycling trips confined to quiet trails designated for bikers. Don't ride along busy streets or in traffic. And by the way, the helmet rule is not an example of "Do as I say . . ." You have to wear your helmet too. Every time. How else can your kid learn?

## BIKE HELMETS

Age-appropriate helmets that meet the government's standards for safety are available for kids of every size. Beware of
helmets that form an "arrow" shape, or are pointy in the back,
since your kid's head will be pushed forward onto his chest by
the seat back. Any helmet that is cracked or damaged in any
way should be considered unsafe and not used by anyone.
For a more exhaustive list of helmet and bike safety rules,
myths, and suggestions, refer to the Child Health Topics section of the American Academy of Pediatrics Web site:
www.aap.org.

As for other riding toys, the helmet rules do not end with
bicycles. Kids riding on scooters, skates, and other wheeled
toys can get hurt. Little kids who are just learning to walk or
ride should ride only on toys that are wide-based, sturdy, and
low enough for the tot to place both feet flat upon the floor. As
your child's balance and motor skills improve, he will gradually be able to steer and learn to use pedals. By the time he is
three, little Mario is probably ripping around on a tricycle and
clamoring for a three-wheeled scooter. Whatever the riding toy,
make sure the device is age-appropriate for your child and that

## EMERGENCY!

If your kid does fall off his bike or another wheeled device, the
same rules as for all other falls apply. If he is unconscious or
not moving, call 911. Watch for signs of a head injury, such as
acting very dazed or inappropriate or repeated vomiting.
Scrapes, bruises, and cuts go hand in hand with kids and
moving vehicles. A broken arm or leg is not unheard of. If you
have any doubts, call your doctor.

safe handling and protective gear are an absolute. No helmet, no toy. Even a toddler should wear a helmet when riding outside, no matter how low or slow she goes; it's a great way to instill a lifesaving habit into your child.

## Drowning

After automobile accidents, the second most common cause of injury-related accidental death among children is drowning. Little kids can drown in as little as an inch of water. Their heads are pretty big and heavy in relation to the body and a curious toddler need only peer over the side of a mop bucket, lose his balance, and wind up upside down and stuck, unable to free his face from the water. Don't keep buckets or other sources of standing water in or around the house. Close the lid of the toilet. Is there a lid on the fish tank? Near larger bodies of water, such as pools, hot tubs, bathtubs, lakes, rivers, and oceans, children should *always* be supervised. Leaving them alone even for "just a second" may have a disastrous outcome. Any pool that may be visited by a child should be surrounded on *all* sides by a gated (and self-latching) fence that is at least four feet high. The side of the house is *not* a fence if there is a door or window in it! Same for the hot tub. Swimming lessons are *not* a substitute for a pool fence.

If your baby or child has found his way into a body of water, hopefully you'll be there to pull him immediately to safety. If he seems to have inhaled quite a bit of water and appears limp, pale, or unconscious, call 911. A child who has submersed himself but is alert, coughing to clear the water from his airways, and is otherwise acting fine, *is* fine. If you are worried, call your pediatrician. A kiddo who is in between, say he is coughing and awake but appears dazed or his breathing is quicker or more labored, needs to be checked out. Call your pediatrician or an ambulance for a ride to the ER. He's most likely okay, but his oxygen levels should be checked and his breathing watched for a little bit. Children may appear fine at first, but then slowly develop more trouble breathing over the next several hours. If you are worried because your child's cough is worsening or he has difficulty breathing, call your doctor right away.

## TOILET LOCKS

They make these locks for the toilet lid, so your kid won't topple in headfirst or go share a drink with the dog. I *did* say that an inch of water was enough to drown a toddler. Even if this does sound a bit neurotic.

## The Bathtub

There is no phone call important enough, no doorbell annoying enough, no deep desire for a cookie great enough, to justify leaving your child alone in the tub for even one second. A baby bath seat is *not* a substitute for supervision. A small child who can sit independently, stand up, and climb out of the bath is *still* at risk of slipping under the water. It takes less than a minute for a child to suffer serious, possibly permanent, injury or even death from being underwater, unable to breathe.

Not only are bathtubs an obvious danger, all that nice-smelling stuff you've dumped in there may pose a special problem. The oils and soaps that turn bath time into fun time can cause direct injury to the lungs. Therefore, if your little one slips under the water, coughs and sputters, and then appears otherwise fine, good. If, however, she seems to have taken a good lungful of bath oil and seems to have increasing coughing or trouble breathing, call your doctor immediately.

And now I've scared you into hosing her off out back every evening. Not my intention. Just bring the phone with you into the bathroom.

## Crib Safety

According to the U.S. Consumer Product Safety Commission (www.cpsc.gov), 97 crib-related deaths (*not* sudden infant death syndrome [SIDS], or crib death) were reported between the years 2002 and 2004. The majority of these tragic events were due to either inappropriate bedding or entrapment due to old or broken crib components or an ill-fitting mattress. Most of the remaining fatalities were due to falls, crib alterations, and strangulation on nearby window cords.

If a used crib was purchased within the last few years, meets all current government safety standards, has never been modified or "repaired," and has no broken, loose, or ill-fitting pieces, it's likely to be okay. Otherwise, you're going shopping. Look at the crib from the eyes of an infant. If there is any possible way to get your head, arms, legs, or body trapped, strangled, cut, pinched, poisoned, or broken, don't use it. If your kid can find a way out, she'll fall, or worse, get trapped between the crib and the wall or another piece of furniture.

Babies go into cribs. Stuffed animals, fluffy blankets, and nice, soft pillows *don't*. Basically, anything that looks soft and inviting is a potential suffocation device. Any blankets in the crib should be thin and either be tightly swaddled around a small infant, or tucked firmly around the mattress and only as high as your wee one's chest. You might consider a nice warm sleeper instead of a blanket if you're feeling a bit nippy.

## Choosing a Crib

When choosing a crib, don't go for aesthetics, think safety. There are a whole mess of rules about choosing and using a crib wisely, all of which are clearly discussed on the American Academy of Pediatrics Web site: www.aap.org/family/inffurn.htm.

Make sure there is nothing on or near the crib with which a baby can become caught or strangle himself. Any crib toys, such as mobiles, need to be up out of reach. The AAP recommends removing any crib toys when a baby is five months old, or has learned to push up onto her hands and knees. Be very careful of nearby window cords and curtains, as they are both potential means of escape as well as agents of suffocation.

If your baby falls from the crib or otherwise injures herself, the rules for managing her injuries and seeking medical care remain the same as for other mechanisms of injury. A baby shouldn't be injured if placed into a properly chosen and correctly used crib. And don't forget that she will, at some point, outgrow her little cage. Before she can sit unsupported,

## Back to Sleep

The recommendation to place infants on their backs to sleep has nearly halved the risk of sudden infant death syndrome (which was pretty rare to begin with, so don't stay up all night watching him!). Placing a baby on his side increases the risk that he can roll to his belly during the night. So he goes on his back. He won't choke on his vomit. When he's old enough to roll about, don't restrain him or force him to lie on his back. He can make his own decision.

the mattress must be lowered, and should be at its lowest point before she can pull to a stand. The AAP wants you to stop using a crib once a kid is thirty-five inches tall. If she can pour herself cereal, she needs a big-girl bed.

## Severe Bleeding

I know this sounds obvious, but in case you are panicking, calm down. If your kiddo climbs on top of the fridge and gets into the knives and has somehow managed to seriously cut himself, get the nearest towel or piece of cloth and apply firm pressure. Do not try to apply a tourniquet or place any instruments into the wound to try to block bleeding blood vessels. Just hold pressure on it until help arrives.

> ### 911!
> If you are seeing severe, spraying blood coming from your child, don't panic. Apply very firm pressure (enough to make him cry) and call 911.

## Electrical Shock

When I was a toddler, I spent an entire afternoon trying to show my mother that my finger hurt. I kept sticking it in her face and saying "Ow." But she couldn't see anything wrong with it and sent me away repeatedly. Finally, after about the tenth "Ow," she followed me, only to find me sticking my finger in the light socket and saying "Ow."

If your kid manages to give himself a little shock, he's most likely fine. Electrical currents travel in lines. They have to start and stop somewhere. Electricity loves to run through water and skin but most commonly with small shocks will travel in a little arc straight in and straight out. This is important, because the life-threatening injuries that occur from an electric shock happen when an electrical current travels into the body and across a vital structure, such as the heart. Sticking your finger in the light socket means the electricity will most likely travel into the finger and out of the finger. This is different from grabbing a live wire with both hands, because then the electricity might travel from one arm to the other, possibly running through the heart. Severe electrical shocks can stop the heart, burn bones and muscles, and cause damage to the kidneys or other organs.

## EMERGENCY!

If your child has suffered what you believe to be a significant shock, first make sure she is moved away from the source of the electrical current. *Do not* grab her if she is still near or stuck to the source of electricity, because you will be shocked as well. Instead, use something that doesn't carry electricity (wood, like a broomstick, is good, as opposed to anything metal or wet, which are great electrical conductors) to push her away from the source of the shock. If she is unconscious or not breathing, call 911. If she is awake and crying, you can relax. If a kid suffers a shock that is significant enough to cause serious injury, but is awake and breathing, nothing bad is likely to happen in the immediate period after the shock and you have time to call your doctor for further instructions.

For most kids, an electric shock means a tiny little jolt from a frayed cord or a socket. These injuries would only extremely rarely be dangerous. A burn may occur from the entry or exit of the electrical shock, but the presence and size of a burn are very poor indicators of the severity of the shock. A severely injured child may have the tiniest of marks, while a larger burn may occur in a child who is well, and vice versa. So, if your little one suffers a minor jolt and appears fine, she is most likely perfectly okay, but you may want to call your pediatrician for anything but the most minor of shocks. For any child who has suffered an electric shock and develops dark or cola-colored urine, your pediatrician needs to know right away.

## Shockproofing

We may be indebted to Ben Franklin for allowing us to stay up past 7 p.m., but keeping your little one safe from man's modern miracle is no easy feat. Especially if he's as curious as I was. Hmm, what would happen if I put this paper clip in *there*? To keep your kid safe, make sure that all electrical cords are in good condition and out of reach. For cords that must be near the ground, make sure they are intact and, when possible, covered with electrical tape or carpeting. A loose, hanging cord can strangle a child, so even an unplugged cord can be a danger. All outlets should be fitted with a childproof plug, although these are pretty easy for a more advanced kid to remove. Outlet plugs should be big enough that a kid can't choke on them. A more extensive outlet cover may slow him down long enough for you to find out why he's so contentedly playing in the other room. Outlets that have plugs running into them should also be concealed with a child-resistant outlet cover. Don't let little kids play with a plug, even when unplugged. It will go into his mouth, get wet, and then zap the heck out of *you*. Avoid using electrical appliances around any body of water, as electricity loves to leap and arc its way across a wet surface. Oh, and don't swim in a thunderstorm, stand with a metal bat in a lightning storm, or climb an electrical tower. I think that covers it.

## Fire

You can always impress your dinner guests with a recipe involving fire. Of course, you can also burn your house down that way. The care of minor burns is covered elsewhere. Unfortunately, injuries due to major fires are rarely confined to small burns. Smoke inhalation and exposure to toxic fumes are the leading causes of injury due to major fires. Little ones, with their rapid respiratory rates, tiny airways, and inability to make a run for it, are especially vulnerable.

Kids can't be expected to know what to do in case of a fire unless someone shows them. Make sure your toddler or young child knows what the smoke alarm is for, what it sounds like, and what to do in case of a fire. If your kid is old enough, you can practice staying low and crawling under the

### 911!

If your house catches on fire, grab your kid and head for the nearest exit. Someone should be calling 911. If your child has suffered any type of burn, especially of the hands, feet, or face, he will need emergency care. Even without any evidence of burn injury, a child who has inhaled smoke or toxic fumes is at risk for severe lung injury. If your child is coughing or having trouble breathing, he needs to be seen immediately. Ditto for a hoarse voice. Call 911. Any soot or ash around the nose and mouth might be a sign of soot and ash in the airways and your kid needs an evaluation.

## SMOKE DETECTORS

According to the CDC, the fifth most common cause of unintentional fatalities in the United States is fire and burns, with children four years and under considered at increased risk. Smoke alarms are invaluable when it comes to protecting your family from a devastating fire. Every floor of the house should have at least one alarm, particularly near your sleeping quarters. Alarms should be tested monthly and the batteries should be changed twice a year. Many people change the batteries when it's time to reset the clocks. I like to "spring forward, fall back, and yell at my husband to change the batteries."

smoke, feeling doors to see if they are hot, and getting out of the nearest window or exit. Teach your kid to roll along the floor to put out the flames if his clothes catch fire, not to run, which can make the fire grow. Make sure an adult can easily open any window guards or locks if needing to escape. Your child's first instinct during a fire will be to hide under a bed or in a closet, so make sure he knows how important it is to get out, not hide. Also make sure you have an assigned meeting place outside where the whole family should gather after leaving the house.

If the fire was pretty small and contained quickly, and your child seems completely well and happy (other than annoyed that his cherries jubilee is on permanent hold), he's most likely totally fine. There is a very good chance that the fire department will be showing up soon and the firemen are well trained in deciding when someone needs an ambulance or a trip to the ER. If the fire department isn't involved and you have any worries, give your pediatrician a call.

## CARBON MONOXIDE DETECTORS

I hope I don't have to tell you that it is a bad idea to light up your charcoal grill in the living room, no matter how miserable the weather. Unfortunately, there are other sources of carbon monoxide, such as stoves and furnaces, that may cause an increase in levels of this odorless, colorless, and potentially fatal gas. Carbon monoxide basically binds to the parts of your red blood cells that carry oxygen and then don't let go, so even though there is oxygen in your lungs, it can't get to the cells of the body. Every house should have at least one carbon monoxide detector, especially near the bedrooms. If the alarm goes off, gather everyone up and head outside, opening doors and windows along the way, and call the fire department. Signs of carbon monoxide poisoning include nausea, sleepiness, and headache, all of which can be confused with the flu, which makes it vitally important that your home be equipped with both smoke *and* carbon monoxide detectors. If a child is exposed to carbon monoxide, oxygen is given to remove the poison from the body and save the oxygen-starved organs, but early recognition is very important.

## Suffocation

Anything that keeps a child from breathing properly can lead to a lack of oxygen, loss of consciousness, and possibly death. Children do, rarely, suffocate or strangulate, most commonly from an accidental hanging or in a bed or crib. If you have followed all the rules for crib safety, you've done a great deal to protect your child. Make sure that your bed and any other beds in the house are positioned in a way that will avoid entrapment of a small child, such as against the wall. Headboards, footboards, and railings should be secure and without any risk of ensnaring a little one. Not only are waterbeds so 1970, but they are potentially dangerous for little kids, who might get stuck between the frame and mattress, or for babies who aren't able to roll or crawl off a moving, gushy surface.

Accidental strangulation is another, tragic, way in which a small child may suffocate. Just use your common sense. Make sure that the string clipping his pacifier to his shirt is short enough to pull on the clothing a bit. Don't wrap him up in a long scarf, or tie his mittens to his jacket with a long piece of string. No playing with plastic bags. Make sure your window treatment cords are child-safe.

If your kid does manage to catch himself around the neck, is quickly freed, and is alert and crying, he's going to be okay. If there are red marks or bruising along the neck, give your doctor a call, but it's unlikely that there is any serious injury. If, however, he is unconscious, not breathing, or having difficulty breathing, remove him from whatever has trapped or suffocated him and call 911 immediately.

## WINDOW CORDS

Babies and small children can become entangled in window cords and easily strangle. Ideally, window coverings should be cordless. Any cords should be short and out of reach. All continuous-loop style cords should be anchored firmly to the ground. Move cribs, beds, toys, and other climbing surfaces far from the window. More information on window and cord safety can be found on the Window Covering Safety Council Web site: www.windowcoverings.org.

## Guns

I'm not actually going to tell you whether a kid who has been shot with a gun requires medical attention. That would be ridiculous. But I will take one moment to rant and rave about gun safety. Children are stupid. They are curious. That is a dangerous combination. No child should be considered gun-safe. If you absolutely insist on having a gun in the home, the gun should be kept in a securely locked location, with the ammunition kept in an entirely separate spot. If your kid has a playdate, don't be embarrassed to ask about any guns in the home. And by the way, a BB gun *can* put your eye out. Ralphie's mom was right.

# going to the emergency room

Well, here we are. If your pediatrician or family doctor thinks it is time for you to take your kid in for an urgent or emergent evaluation, you should listen. It is better to be safe than sorry. There is actually a very good chance that you will be sent right back home with nothing more than discharge papers. They say a picture paints a thousand words, and laying an eyeball on a kid for a nanosecond can tell volumes more than three hours of telephone calls. Sometimes that is all your doctor wants: an eyeball. Other times your kid might actually need care. This chapter will let you know what awaits, in the hope that a little preparation will go a long way toward keeping your visit as pleasant as it can possibly be.

## The Logistics

### Choosing a Facility

In case of a true emergency, the best emergency room is the closest one. However, if you have the luxury of choice when it comes to selecting a care center, there are a couple of things you should think about.

First and foremost is with which hospital does your doctor have a relationship? Most pediatricians are "affiliated" with a hospital within the community and will send their patients there. The reasons for selecting a hospital with which to have a relationship are many, often influenced by where a doctor has trained and whom he knows. Having a relationship with the hospital and its doctors and services allows your doctor to keep tabs on what is happening and remain in close contact with the managing team during your child's hospital stay.

A second consideration when choosing a hospital or ER is whether the hospital has a designated pediatric ER or doctors specifically trained in pediatrics and pediatric emergency medicine, like me. Some ERs will have pediatric specialists and others will have doctors trained in general emergency medicine, meaning they have some pediatric training but see patients of all ages. The much bigger question you should ask yourself is how comfortable is this hospital in treating ill or injured kids? If they see one kid a year, maybe not so good, but if the doctors and nurses care for children on a regular basis, they're likely to be quite capable at handling anything.

If you have any doubt about which hospital or ER to choose, let your pediatrician guide you. She can make it much

## CHOOSING A HOSPITAL

It is a good idea to ask your pediatrician which hospital you will be sent to in an emergency. Find out exactly where the hospital is and make a quick scouting trip, to see where the main and emergency entrances are, find a parking garage, and gain a general idea about the campus. A little familiarization might go a long way if you ever find yourself trying to navigate a medical center when panicked or stressed.

easier for you not only by calling ahead and letting the doctors know that your kid will be arriving but also by giving the staff valuable additional medical history. If your pediatrician isn't available and you have to make a choice on your own, try to find out which center sees the most kids in that town. A hospital designated for children or one with a pediatric wing would likely be preferable to one that doesn't treat or hospitalize kids. Don't be swayed by which hospital looks the prettiest or has the shortest wait. Try to choose the place that will best serve your child.

## Arriving

Once you've gotten to the hospital, what happens next depends on your child's condition and complaint. Whether a kid comes by ambulance or by family car, the sickest kids will be seen first, not the ones accompanied by the most noise and bright lights. Once a kid arrives at the hospital, he is "triaged," meaning that a quick assessment of his age, vital signs, and complaint are made and he is assigned a triage category. This category allows us to group kids by severity of illness or injury so that the sickest kids get seen first and the rest in a somewhat orderly fashion. A nurse or other hospital worker should listen to your concerns and create a hospital chart, documenting all relevant medical history and your child's vital signs. Be sure to provide all past medical history at this point, because some conditions may seem irrelevant to you but can significantly change the gravity of your child's condition. Please report any medications, including over-the-counter drugs, that your little one is currently (or was recently) taking, including dosages.

## Waiting

If the ER is empty (unlikely) or your kid is deemed high priority by triage category, you and your little one may be swept right into an examining area. What is more likely, however, is that after being triaged, your family will be sent to the waiting area. If you are lucky enough to be in a center that treats lots of children, there may be cartoons and playthings. Hopefully you had time to grab a couple of favorite toys or books to keep your kid occupied. I'm sorry to say that the average waiting time for all emergency rooms in the United States is currently in excess of three hours. How long you will have to wait varies dramatically and is dependent on a multitude of factors. If the ER is pretty empty and rooms are available and the other patients aren't very sick, you may be in and out in an hour. An hour is, by the way, light speed in hospital time. On the other hand, if you arrive and the ER is empty but there is a critically ill or dying child commanding everyone's attention, you will have to wait until someone has the time to attend to you. Parents can get pretty angry waiting to be seen in an emergency room. It can be very frustrating to see patients who arrived after them called first or children who appear to be very well taken immediately

### WAITING IN THE ER

Your wait to be seen in the ER may vary from minutes to hours. Depending on your child's condition, food or drink may be encouraged or forbidden. Please ask the triage nurse if it is okay to feed your little one. You would hate to get to the exam area and find out that those vending machine crackers he ate are going to cost you four extra hours of time waiting for his tummy to empty!

back. Please, please try to remember that many factors determine the order in which patients are seen, and you may not have a complete perspective. It is possible that seven ambulances from a house fire just pulled in out back or that well-appearing child actually has a history of cancer.

## Getting to a Room

Yay! The nurse has finally called you into an exam area! You're halfway there. But just because you've been called into a room doesn't mean you will be seen immediately. The workflow in the ER is such that beds are filled as they become available and doctors and nurses work as hard and as fast as they can to get to new patients. However, this means that we may still be finishing up something else or another patient is requiring our attention. The same rules about waiting apply whether you are in the waiting room or in an examination area. Try to be patient. Know that we know you are there. Follow instructions regarding food and drink. We want to deal with your problem as quickly as possible.

While you might think that the doctors sitting at the desk writing on charts are doing nothing more than sipping coffee and chatting, that is not the case. They might not actually work in the ER. Some of those doctors doing "nothing" might be consulting physicians stopping by to say hi to their patients. Some could be medical students who have been forbidden to see another patient until the attending can disposition their current one.

## The Real Party Begins

Quick! Close that drawer you were snooping in! Here comes the doctor. Depending on the institution, you may be seen by a nurse practitioner (NP), a physician's assistant (PA), a medical student, a resident, or a supervising doctor. Don't be upset if the first person you see is not the doctor in charge of the ER. Because of the workload in most emergency rooms, physician "extenders" such as NPs and PAs often see lower-acuity patients to help keep the flow moving. These individuals are well trained and practice only under the supervision of a physician, whom you may or may not physically see. In a training hospital, medical students and junior physicians are often the first to evaluate patients. This can be a real bonus, because one supervising doctor can oversee and advise six or seven junior members much faster than he can do the work himself. For example, if the supervising doctor were to see the patient without a junior-level assistant, he would have to see the patient, write the medication and laboratory orders, make multiple phone calls to radiology or the pediatrician or a consultant, write up the chart, follow up on results, repeat phone calls, and finally write up the discharge papers or arrange a hospital admission. For each patient. In a smaller hospital, this works okay, but when the flow of patients increases, not having assistance can bring the workload to a grinding halt. So embrace your medical student, because she is the one who is going to get you through the system as quickly and painlessly as possible.

Once your kid has been seen and a plan of action decided upon, what happens next can range from absolutely nothing and a discharge form to a myriad of trips around the hospital, tests and radiology studies, and possibly admission to the hospital or transfer to another institution. Making a diagnosis and deciding on the best course of treatment are not always easy and can sometimes take hours. Once we have gathered our facts, the decision to send a child home or admit him to the hospital is made and plans can be carried out. If your pediatrician sent you to the hospital, he should be aware of the treatment plan, but feel free to double-check at the hospital that your pediatrician has been called.

## WHAT IS THE HOLDUP?

It may seem like everything takes forever in the ER and sometimes it does. If your hospital is lucky enough to have a designated laboratory or radiology suite for the emergency room's use, fantastic! But there still might be fifteen or twenty X-rays in the queue before your kid's. The lab might be backed up. It might take a half hour to reach a consulting physician. All these delays add up, but believe me, as frustrated as you are, we are too. We honestly aren't trying to torture you.

## Medical Procedures

### Preparing for a Procedure

In an attempt to demystify some of the workings of the ER, I'll try to describe several of the more common procedures that are performed in an emergency setting. While many of these sound scary, and none are without some degree of risk, these procedures are both routine and necessary when deciding whether a child is truly in need of certain medications or further treatment.

Unfortunately, there may be times when a blood test or other procedure should be performed, which is likely to make your little one cry. Babies and kids don't like to be held down, let alone poked with a needle. Given the choice, I don't know many who are going to sit still and cooperate during an uncomfortable moment. As difficult as it is to watch your child experience pain and discomfort, a couple of thoughts may be helpful. First, we don't enjoy it. I promise. Second, as cruel as we may look, strapping your child to a "papoose" board, wrapping him in a sheet "mummy style," or even (rarely and only when I have to) lying across his thrashing body (this usually applies more to drunk teenagers covered in vomit), properly restraining a fighting child gives the greatest chance of performing the procedure in a fast, efficient, and successful manner.

## NPO

The acronym *NPO* stands for *non per os*, which is Latin for "nothing by mouth." Prior to receiving sedation, except in extreme emergent circumstances, a patient must be NPO for a standardized period of time, which varies from institution to institution but generally means at least two hours for clear liquids and six to eight hours for food. The reason for this is that a person is so relaxed during sedation that stomach contents could wind up in the lungs, with serious consequences. Nothing by mouth means just that. Nothing. If you give your kid a sip of juice in the waiting room, that is something and it counts. Ask the triage nurse if your child can eat and drink while waiting, and if he eats a cookie or drinks a soda, fess up when asked.

If your child needs to undergo a procedure, in most circumstances it is the parent's right to stay by his side. As long as you aren't interfering with the medical staff or making the child more anxious, having a parent in the room during a procedure can not only help calm the child, but also reassure the parent that the medical staff is doing their very best to ensure little Sam's health and safety.

> ## It's All in the Restraint
> If you want to be involved in the proper restraint of your child, please feel free, but you need to mean it. Too many parents cave at the last minute, when a sudden movement by a child results in a failed attempt at the procedure. It is absolutely okay to step back and ask someone else to be the "big meanie."

On the same note, if you don't want to be in the room when your child is having a blood draw or other procedure, either because you can't stand to watch little Susie cry *or* because you tend to pass out and throw up at the sight of blood, don't feel bad about stepping out for a cup of coffee. Go get your beverage, and your kid will be waiting for you when you return.

## Needle Pokes

Quite a few kids who come to the ER escape without a poke or a stick. Unfortunately, however, blood draws and intravenous lines (IVs) are pretty common procedures in the emergency room. Little kids have little blood vessels, are often wrapped in a layer of vessel-hiding chub, and they don't exactly cooperate when faced with a needle. Several attempts are sometimes made before blood can be successfully drawn or an IV is well placed. Whether the procedure is successful is dependent not just on the skill of the person performing it, but also on the kid's condition, age, and body type, the shape of the moon, my daily horoscope, and so on. In other words, the best IV nurse in the world may not be able to get a line in a kid when a first-time attempt by a medical student succeeds. It is a little about skill and a lot about luck. Try not to become upset if a few tries are needed before success. Depending on the severity of a child's illness, obtaining intravenous access may be lifesaving, in which case attempts at IV placement continue until successful. On the other hand, if a kid is more stable, it is okay to ask for a short break to give your little one a chance to calm down and have a rest if several attempts have been fruitless.

In case you are worried about where the IV is going to go, the optimal spot for an IV is where it can be successfully placed. Hands and feet, arms and ankles are all options. Sometimes we will place an IV into the more superficial veins of the neck, which sounds scary but is very safe. In little babies, the easiest vein to find may be on the scalp. An IV placed into a scalp vein does *not* go through the skull or in any way come near the brain. For more difficult cases or in children who need more advanced forms of blood vessel access, a central line, or very large IV, may be placed into one of the major blood vessels of the body. And don't become worried that your child will perish because of a lack of an IV. In an emergency we can place a special IV right into the bone, which sounds really scary but is actually a very easy and foolproof way of getting lifesaving medicines into a child.

## The Spinal Tap

If a baby or child comes to the ER and we are worried about meningitis, a lumbar puncture, or spinal tap, will be performed. It sounds cruel, but a spinal tap is something done every day, sometimes several times a day, on babies and children, even tiny little newborns. As frightening as this sounds, it is very simple and has a very low risk of any complications when performed correctly. After cleaning the lower back with antiseptic solution, a very tiny needle is placed into the space between the backbones where some of the spinal fluid sits. The spinal cord ends well above this space and there is no risk of paralysis. After less than a teaspoon of fluid is taken, the needle is removed, a little bandage is placed over the site, and it's done. Occasionally there might be a little trouble finding that tiny space or a little blood vessel might get hit during the procedure. Neither of these will injure a child in any way; it just makes our job a little more difficult. In older children, numbing medicine is used before inserting the spinal needle. In babies and smaller children, whether an injection of numbing medicine is used is dependent on several factors such as the child's age and size, how awake he is, and so on. However, it is perfectly acceptable to request that some numbing cream be placed on the child's skin, no matter his age, prior to the procedure if the staff has not already done so. Nobody wants to hear that their child needs a spinal tap, but remember that the complications of meningitis include blindness, deafness, developmental delay, and possibly even death.

## X-Rays

If your kid needs an X-ray, whether you are going to be allowed in the room and able to assist the technicians is dependent upon the institution. Feel free to ask about how many pictures will be taken and whether a lead apron will be provided to protect your kid's privates and other radiation-sensitive organs. Once the X-rays have been taken, you'll probably be sent back to your assigned room in the ER; however, you may have to go back a few times if the doctors feel additional views or films are needed. Most emergency rooms now view X-rays on a computer, rather than the old-fashioned "hard copy" of the past, meaning that you may not be able to take an X-ray home with you. However, most hospital medical records departments will be happy to provide a copy of any studies for you to have or to take to your pediatrician's office. You just have to call them during regular business hours and they may charge you a small administrative fee.

## CT Scans

A computerized tomography examination, or CT scan, is a fantastic way of looking inside the head and body. CT scans are great for evaluating injuries to the brain and for letting us look at the organs. An MRI scan is a much more detailed test but is generally not available on an emergent basis, so most physicians rely on a CT for an emergency evaluation of many injuries and illnesses.

A CT scanner is shaped like a big ring, with a moving bed that slides in and out. For a CT scan to be adequate, a patient must not be moving, which is unfortunate when dealing with kids. In some centers the technicians are very good at calming a little one and can obtain a scan without medications. However, in many centers, trying to coax a squirming child into a position of absolute stillness for five minutes is too labor- and time-intensive. In addition, if a kid wakes up or begins to move during the study, it will have to be repeated, meaning additional radiation exposure. Because of these reasons, many hospitals will choose to sedate a child who is too young to follow directions and remain motionless.

The medications used to calm a kid for a CT scan vary from hospital to hospital and are for the most part extremely safe. The biggest concern for most kids is making sure that they don't get so tired and relaxed that they forget to breathe effectively. Therefore, a child undergoing sedation for any procedure will often be hooked up to monitors to evaluate his heart rate and oxygen levels and may receive additional oxygen until fully awake. After the CT scan is over, your child should slowly wake up and return to normal over the next hour or so, maybe faster. Once she is awake and alert, the nurse can remove the monitors and she can once again move freely about.

## RADIATION

The fear of exposing your child to excessive levels of radiation is a reasonable one. Regular X-rays and CT scans expose patients to radiation. But there is also natural radiation all around, so living in a brick house exposes you to radiation. The more important question is how much total radiation is received? A regular X-ray is actually quite low in radiation, while CT scans expose one to higher doses. Some hospitals are able to use modern CT scanning technology, which allows the level of radiation used to be adjusted for a child's age and weight. It is prudent to question the need for radiographic testing when discussing your child's condition with her doctor. On the other hand, CT scanning, when performed appropriately, can be lifesaving. We must always consider a risk-benefit ratio. A CT scan is necessary when we are worried about a child, and recommended against when felt to be unnecessary. The very small increased risk from receiving more radiation over a lifetime does not trump the need to save a life today. Feel free to ask a doctor why he is choosing an imaging study that requires radiation, as opposed to one that doesn't. Sometimes there is a reasonable alternative and other times there simply isn't. Please know that these decisions are not made arbitrarily, and we really do want to do right by *your* kid.

## The End

If you actually read this book the whole way through and you aren't one of my parents, good for you! You are now more educated and better prepared than any other parent on your block. A few reminders for you:

- Kids are resilient.
- Parental instinct is not a myth.
- An ounce of prevention is worth a ton of cure.

So relax, grab some sunscreen and a hat, and take your kid outside so that you can properly enjoy this wonderful ride called parenting. Good luck!

———■———

# index

# about the author

Despite receiving a D in Library Sciences at the age of ten, Dr. Lara Zibners persevered in her academic studies, graduating cum laude from the Ohio State University School of Medicine. She then completed both a residency in pediatrics and a fellowship in pediatric emergency medicine at Nationwide Children's Hospital in Columbus, Ohio, and is currently board certified in both general pediatrics and pediatric emergency medicine. After finishing her training, she was awarded the position of assistant professor of pediatric emergency medicine at Mount Sinai Hospital in New York City. In 2006, Dr. Zibners relocated to Great Britain with her husband. Currently living in London, she divides her professional time as an author, speaker, and emergency room pediatrician between London and New York. You can visit her Web site at www.drzibners.com.